Homoeopathic First Aid

Homoeopathic First Aid

Twenty useful medicines for day-to-day problems

Dr Anne M. Clover

THORSONS PUBLISHING GROUP

First published 1990

British Library Cataloguing in Publication Data

Clover, Anne M.
  Homoeopathic first aid.
  1. Medicine. Homoeopathy. Remedies
  I. Title
  615.532

ISBN 0 7225 2107 3

Published by Thorsons Publishers Limited, Wellingborough, Northamptonshire NN8 2RQ, England

Typeset by Burns & Smith Ltd., Derby

Printed in Great Britain by William Collins Sons & Co. Ltd, Glasgow

10 9 8 7 6 5 4 3 2

Contents

Acknowledgements

I thank Becky Houlden for her skilful cartoons and Dr Michael Jenkins for his suggestions on the contents of this book.

Introduction

In recent years there has been a steady increase in the number of people seeking homoeopathic treatment. Those of us who practise in hospitals with departments specializing in this form of therapy and colleagues working in other situations have experienced this trend. At the same time we have had many more requests from groups of people seeking talks introducing the basic principles of homoeopathic medicine and how it can play a part in first aid. This book is intended to help meet the need for such information. I hope it will support the interest of people already using homoeopathic medicines themselves and encourage others to begin to try, for their own first aid needs, medicines that for decades have been found safe and effective.

The first two chapters will introduce the ideas on which homoeopathic medicine is based. The next five chapters will refer to particular medical situations with suggestions of homoeopathic medicines that may contribute to their treatment. The final chapter will include reflections on the usefulness of an increasing knowledge of homoeopathy in first aid.

The aim throughout this book is to assist home prescribing for day-to-day problems. The data considered are therefore presented with an emphasis on particular features that can guide prescribing in specific situations requiring first aid. They are not intended to be a comprehensive review of the type found in detailed homoeopathic materia medica.

The twenty medicines to which these chapters will refer and

their source materials are as follows:

Aconite, from the plant also known as monkshood.

Antimonium tartaricum, from the tartrate of antimony and potash.

Argentum nitricum, from silver nitrate.

Arnica, from the plant *Arnica montana* or leopard's bane, found particularly in the Swiss Alps.

Arsenicum album, from the white oxide of arsenic.

Belladonna, from the plant *Atropa belladonna* or the deadly nightshade.

Bryonia, from the root of the plant also known as white bryony.

Cantharis, derived from an insect, the Spanish fly.

Chamomilla, from the plant of that name.

Gelsemium, from the bark of the root of *Gelsemium sempervirens*.

Kali bichromicum, from a bichromate of potash.

Ledum, from the plant *Ledum palustre*, also known as wild rosemary.

Mercurius solubis, a mercury preparation.

Natrum muriaticum, an extract of common salt, sodium chloride.

Nux vomica, from the seeds of the plant also known as poison nut.

Phosphorus, from red phosphorus.

Pulsatilla, from the plant also known as *Anemone pratensis*, the wind flower.

Rhus toxicodendron, from the leaves of the plant also known as poison oak and closely related to poison ivy.

Staphisagria, from the seeds of *Delphinium staphisagria* or stavesacre.

> **Symphytum**, from the fresh-root stock of *Symphytum*
> *officinale* or comfrey.

It will be quickly recognized that many of these source
materials are highly poisonous in their crude state. When used
in homoeopathic medicines they have been very carefully
extracted and prepared so that they are presented in highly
dilute forms which are safe for use. All the subsequent
discussions in this book will refer to using these extracts
prepared by homoeopathic manufacturing pharmacists and
nowhere imply use of the crude source materials.

CHAPTER 1

What is Homoeopathy?

Many of the people who request homoeopathic medicine are trying it as a new form of treatment for themselves and are unfamiliar with its basic ideas. They therefore often ask 'what is homoeopathy?' A short answer is to describe it as a safe and effective form of medicine found useful over many decades for a wide range of medical needs. This description makes homoeopathy sound no different from many other forms of therapy. So what are its special characteristics?

When this question is asked today, many people refer immediately to the small doses of the medicine often used by homoeopathic prescribers. The term 'homoeopathic' has even crept into popular vocabulary being used, for example, to refer to weak tea. This is a common misuse of the term. It is true that homoeopaths may use small doses, a fact we will look at further in the next chapter. But this is not the precise implication of the term homoeopathy which, rather than referring to the size of the doses given, actually summarizes the way in which they are selected.

A homoeopathic medicine is one that in appropriate doses in a test situation could provoke in people symptoms similar to those it can treat when used in therapy. It is sometimes loosely described as using likes for likes, or having a hair of the dog that bit you. It is an idea closely related to the use of vaccines, where highly refined extracts of disease-causing agents are used in the preventive therapy of the diseases they can cause. This principle is applied in homoeopathy to help seek medical stimuli for a wide range of disorders from causes as various as infection or injury, wear and tear or anxiety. It is often described as the 'similia principle'.

An example will illustrate this basic tenet of homoeopathic prescribing. When peeling onions many people produce tears and a watery nasal discharge. It is a very familiar reaction that most people know well. We know too that the symptoms of a common cold can include similar watering eyes and runny nose. This means that onions can cause effects on people similar to those that occur in common colds. Applying the similia principle means that an extract of onion suitably

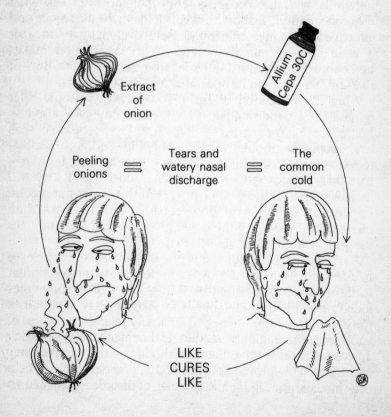

Extract of onion

Peeling onions ≡ Tears and watery nasal discharge ≡ The common cold

LIKE CURES LIKE

prepared can be used to treat people suffering from colds. The agent that can cause similar effects can be used, in a suitably prepared form, to treat them when they occur in a disease. Another easily recognized example is the use of extracts of pollens and grasses in the treatment of hay fever. Again, a substance capable of producing symptoms is used in a specially prepared form for their treatment.

The possibility of using medicines in this way has been known from very early times. Even the writings of Hippocrates make some reference to it. But its implications and use were not developed until the late eighteenth and early nineteenth centuries. Modern homoeopathy owes a great deal to the pioneer work of Samuel Hahnemann, who was born in Meissen, Saxony in 1755 and subsequently trained as a doctor and chemist. His biography relates how he noted that a medicine called cinchona, used in his day to treat malaria, could produce, in people who did not have the infection, symptoms similar to those seen with the disease. It was his personal observation that cinchona could either treat the effects of malaria, or provoke similar symptoms, that led him to do a lot of detailed research work and writing describing his findings. This work, all founded on the observation of the similia principle, has become the basis of modern homoeopathic medicine.

Hahnemann's writings show that for him three questions were very important for the pursuit of any therapy. He repeatedly argued that for all therapy we need to ask, first, what is happening in a disease process; second, what are the properties of medicines; and third, how therefore can such medicines be safely and effectively used in therapy? It is a logical three-stage sequence seeking a knowledge of diseases, then of medicines and finally of how to relate the first two steps for treatment.

While pursuing these studies, Hahnemann always observed two other points fundamental to all homoeopathic treatment. The first is that disease processes, their causes and effects, are always individual to the person experiencing them. This means that even when treating children in a measles epidemic he would say that you need to treat not measles, but a form of measles. Even in epidemics individual patients show particular forms of the diseases concerned. The second principle is that all visible, measurable effects of diseases are due to hidden causes that need taking into account for adequate therapy. These two principles, that disease is always an individual experience to the patient and that its visible effects are indications of hidden processes, remain very important for accurate homoeopathic prescribing today.

We live now in an era when it is generally accepted that personal details, including hidden psychological factors, are relevant to disease. It is worth noting that Hahnemann was writing about such awareness at least 50 years before Sigmund Freud's pioneer work made him famous and led to the wider acknowledgement that hidden psychological pressures are relevant to all aspects of health and disease. The acceptance of such insight has been further facilitated in recent years through the growth of research concerning the psychological factors in many, some people would say all, diseases. We know now that the body is an energy system, that even hard bones are made up by patterns of energy behaving in a manner that makes them appear and function as solid forms. This awareness makes it much easier to accept that the energies of thought and emotion not only can contribute to our physical processes, but actually do so in every moment of our existence, in health and disease. The physical body is not separate from the psychological processes we experience. Both our psyche and soma are aspects of the energy complex that constitutes our being.

Such insight is employed in homoeopathic medicine today when, applying the similia principle, we seek to use a medicine that not only relates to the measurable physical effects of diseases, but also refers to the psychological processes experienced by the person seeking help. Often in a first-aid situation there is an initial emphasis on the particular physical effects of disease or injury. But, with any treatment we offer, it is also helpful if we can be aware of the psychological reactions. This can be particularly important when individual patients are shocked psychologically as well as physically by an accident or disease. A homoeopathic medicine relevant to the emotional and physical aspects of the distress can be a very useful part of the treatment offered. At the same time, it may assist the therapeutic ideal of seeking more understanding of the processes involved in diseases as well as easing their effects.

Such an approach, it may be argued, is important for at least two reasons. First, it may help us avoid some of the factors that can provoke disease. Second, it can help us learn more about ourselves and enable better use of our healthy organism. Greater understanding of any structure can help us both avoid difficulties and use it more extensively. We may use a car, a video-recorder or a word processor. With all such machines more knowledge of what damages them, as well as how to use the facilities they offer, will extend their use. Our human bodies are similar; and, if we will, we can use an experience of disease to learn through it whilst also seeking medicines for relief of unpleasant effects.

Homoeopathy is one of the forms of medicine that can be used for both of these aspects of therapy. It is a method of delivering a medical stimulus to help restore health and, with its emphasis on prescribing for individual needs, is particularly useful for encouraging detailed questioning of the processes involved.

Basically, therefore, homoeopathy is one of the methods for choosing a medicine to help relieve disease and restore health. It is a system of prescribing. It includes careful evaluation of the effects of a disease process and then the selection of a particular medicine to assist healing.

For many diseases the body has an inbuilt defence mechanism that, in perhaps a few days, will gradually overcome and re-establish a more healthy state. These are usually termed acute diseases. Examples are influenza and mumps. For other diseases, the body finds this more difficult and the process is naturally much longer lasting and described as chronic. A common example is some forms of rheumatoid arthritis. For both acute and chronic diseases an appropriate medicine may assist the body's healing mechanism. Even if diseases are likely to be naturally self-limiting, it may help a lot if that process is encouraged. When a child has measles both the patient and his or her family will appreciate a speeding-up of the healing process.

The learning about diseases that has to accompany the development of effective therapy has made us increasingly aware that many factors influence its course. Even when infectious organisms such as influenza viruses are implicated, other factors are also relevant. When such infection comes into a home, some people catch it, others do not. Personal vulnerability or resistance can vary greatly for many reasons, reminding us that there is no single cause for disease developing or being resisted. We are increasingly learning that the wide range of diseases we experience can be provoked by causes as various as bacteria and business stress, injury and personal insult. Just as diseases can have many causal factors, similarly various forms of therapy may be required. Hence the advantages of 'complementary medicine', a term used increasingly today to refer to various forms of medical practice that can usefully work together to assist healing.

Homoeopathy is a form of therapy aptly termed complementary. It can be used in conjunction with other appropriate forms of treatment if these are also required. Common examples are the use of homoeopathic prescriptions by people also adjusting their diet, continuing psychotherapy, having surgery or taking other forms of medicine. First aid is a particularly useful example of the complementary role of homoeopathic medicines. If someone has an injury they will obviously need local attention to the wound and dressings as well as medicines that may help their general response. If the injury is severe enough to require surgery, homoeopathic medicines rightly used may help a person to prepare for and recover from the operation. Here the homoeopathic medicines are aptly termed complementary.

The selection of appropriate lines of therapy is clearly important. None of us want to miss out on any aid that can be safely effective. This ideal is important in any treatment situation, including first aid. We make an assessment and advise the form of treatment that according to our experience we expect to help. Any prescriber or helper advises in the light of his particular training. Whether the treatment comes from hospital staff, a person specially trained in first aid, or from a parent helping a child ill at home, it is offered from a basis of personal knowledge of measures that can assist. Such training is clearly very important. So too is a readiness to ask for additional help if the adviser concerned finds the needs are more than they can safely handle. First aid is what the term implies and may lead to a request for additional help in due course. This is very important and as relevant to homoeo-pathic help in first aid as it is for any form of treatment. Hence the emphasis placed on it in this first chapter before we move onto a consideration of homoeopathic medicines that can be used in the therapy of particular disorders.

The selection of the form of a homoeopathic medicine for use leads naturally to the questions about the strength and frequency of the doses. At meetings to discuss homoeopathy and particularly on its use for home first aid, these questions are frequently asked. We will look at them in the next chapter when, as if following Hahnemann's three-stage approach, we turn our attention to the nature of homoeopathic medicines before leading on from this to consider specific prescriptions for particular first aid needs.

CHAPTER 2

Homoeopathic Medicines

The range of sources for homoeopathic medicines is vast. It includes plant materials, minerals, snake venoms, cat or dog hair, extracts of chemical compounds and bacterial products. Applying the similia principle introduced in the previous chapter means that suitably prepared extracts of many agents capable of producing effects in human beings can be used to assist the treatment of similar effects occurring in diseases. Hence the wide range of source materials for homoeopathic medicines. Since Hahnemann developed the application of the similia principle over 100 years ago, the use of the medicines he researched has been extended and many new ones introduced by his successors.

Hahnemann's work included devising methods for the deliberate testing of agents to clarify their effects on the human body. This involved relatively healthy people taking small doses of substances for long enough to illustrate their effects but without causing harm. Hahnemann organized such tests as scientific experiments with careful instructions on how they should be carried out and their results recorded. The tests became known as 'provings' and the volunteer testers as 'provers'. The data they produced formed his *Materia Medica*, that is the prescribing manuals. Provings have continued since Hahnemann's initial work and are still done today. Naturally the technique has been refined as time has gone on, but the basic idea of testing medicines for their possible effects, and then applying the results in prescribing remains a cornerstone of homoeopathic medicine today.

The similia principle also implies that toxicology, or the recorded effects of accidental poisonings, can also at times yield data applicable in homoeopathic practice. An example of this occurred when a well-known homoeopathic practitioner and writer on the subject accidentally absorbed a small amount of venom that had previously been extracted from a poisonous snake. Although the dose was not fatal, it was sufficient to produce some of its characteristic effects. The story is told that as he recovered he saw the events as a proving of the effects of the venom and demanded that his family write down an account of the experience. Since then an extract of the venom, known as *Lachesis*, has been widely used for symptoms as various as menopausal hot flushes and asthma.

A more familiar application of modern toxicology in homoeopathic prescribing comes from petroleum products. It is known that handling them in everyday life can provoke skin eruptions in sensitive people. In homoeopathic practice an extract of petroleum has often been useful in certain forms of eczema.

These illustrations have already referred to medicines from sources as various as reptile venom and oil. Today there are over 2500 substances that have been prepared as homoeopathic medicines. Of these over 60 per cent are from botanical sources. Well-known examples are extracts of belladonna, or deadly nightshade, and aconite or monkshood. Many other medicines are derived from mineral sources; an example is *Arsenicum album*, from white arsenic. A smaller number of homoeopathic medicines derive from animal products, examples being *Lachesis*, the extract of snake venom referred to earlier, and *Cantharis* from the insect known as Spanish fly. Plants, trees and minerals are the sources for the majority of homoeopathic medicines. Many have been used for several decades; others have been added recently. With continuing research in various countries the list is increasing all the time.

Having considered the sources of homoeopathic medicines

we move on to look at the size of the doses. The ideal of using small doses when prescribing homoeopathic medicines was introduced by Hahnemann and continued by his successors. He argued for using the smallest possible dose of a medicine to produce the required therapeutic effects without harm. Hahnemann obtained his degree as a doctor in 1779, a time when large doses of strongly acting medicines were often used with consequent widespread problems from side-effects. It is clear from his own writings, and those of his biographer, that Hahnemann's observations of these problems led to his insistence on using minimal doses of medicines to assist healing as harmlessly as possible. In pursuit of this ideal Hahnemann developed the use of the highly reduced doses of medicine for which homoeopathy is now well known.

The reduction of doses of medicines, pioneered by Hahnemann and continued by his successors, comprises serial dilutions and vigorous agitation of the product at each stage in the preparation. Substances naturally soluble are first dissolved in an alcohol–water mixture to give the crude extract known as a mother tincture. This is then used for the preparation of progressively reduced doses. The reduction Hahnemann pioneered was on a 1:10 or 1:100 scale known respectively as the decimal or centesimal range. Most of Hahnemann's work employed preparations on the centesimal scale. It comprised taking one drop of the medicinal extract and mixing it with 99 drops of diluted alcohol. This solution was then 'succussed', that is vigorously shaken and recurrently thumped down onto a firm surface for a specified time. The first stage led to a 1C preparation. One drop of this, with another 99 drops of diluted alcohol and again succussed, led to the 2C, the second centesimal preparation. The process continued, with dilution and succussion at each stage, to the required degree of reduction. Much of Hahnemann's work was with 30C preparations. That is, dilution and succussion of the mother tincture on the centesimal scale 30 times. For preparations on the decimal scale the sequence was similar but employed 1 drop of medicine with 9 drops of diluted

Homoeopathic medicines

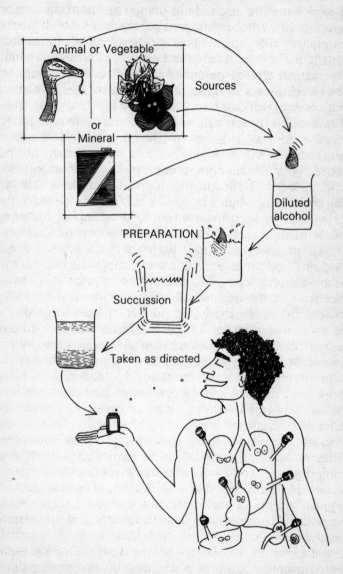

Animal or Vegetable

or

Mineral

Sources

Diluted alcohol

PREPARATION

Succussion

Taken as directed

alcohol for the 1:10 reduction at each stage. For substances that were naturally insoluble in diluted alcohol Hahnemann also devised a method of first grinding them down with precise amounts of milk sugar. This process, called trituration, gradually made them soluble and capable of further handling in the manner already described for medicinal solutions.

The development of these practices must have involved a vast amount of work for Hahnemann and his colleagues. They had minimal technical aids in his day, and he required fresh glassware for each stage in the process. Hahnemann continued to use these highly reduced doses throughout his practice. They remain an important aspect of homoeopathic medicine today. Hahnemann observed that these reduced doses not only continued to assist healing, but also led to the improvement of symptoms without side-effects or upsetting patients in the process. He wrote copiously throughout his years of practice, recording both the techniques he was developing and the effects he saw in patients he treated.

Such observations led Hahnemann into progressive clarification of his understanding of diseases and how they can be treated. His three-fold pursuit of knowledge of the process contributing to diseases, of medicines and then of effective therapy can be seen running all through his reports of his work. By his latter years, after observing and recording the effects of the medicines he used, he deduced that the processes of dilution and succussion of medicines not only reduced unwanted effects, but progressively disrupted medicines releasing energies contained in them but previously veiled by their gross form. These previously hidden resources, he argued, were particularly effective in stimulating the body's own defence mechanisms against disease. He deduced that the reduction exposed more powerful aspects of the medicines which he then termed 'potencies'. The process of preparation was similarly termed 'potentization'.

These terms are still in regular use today. We continue to refer to the potentization of mother tincture preparations, that is the original solution of a medicine, and the prescription of, for instance, 6C or 30C potencies implying medicines diluted and succussed on the centesimal scale 6 or 30 times respectively. The preparation of such medicines today is performed by manufacturers whose techniques are regulated by the legislation of their particular countries.

Medicines produced in this way today can be obtained from many chemists, health food stores, or direct from the manufacturer's own outlets. They can be prescribed by doctors willing to advise homoeopathic medicine either privately or, in Britain, within the National Health Service. Most of the homoeopathic medicines widely used today can also be bought 'over-the-counter' without prescription. This means that they can usually be readily obtained by people wishing to have their own stock of a few well-chosen homoeopathic medicines for home use.

This brings us to the need for some guidance on the dosage of these medicines. Subsequent chapters will refer to the names of particular forms of homoeopathic medicines likely to assist with specific medical needs. To use these or other homoeopathic medicines we need to consider three points: the strength of medicine to be used, how often to take it, and the means of taking it. In short, we need to consider the strength, timing and method for using these medicines.

For first-aid purposes 6C or 30C potencies of homoeopathic medicines are widely used. The suggestions for prescribing in this book will refer to 30C preparations, but if these are not available a 6C could be used. Advice on how often to repeat prescriptions will be given for the particular problems discussed. An additional general guide is that for acute, that is recently occurring problems, a short course of the 30C strength is appropriate. For accidental injuries or for infections an example would be one tablet of the 30C strength of an appropriate medicine 1 or 2 hourly for three doses, and then assess the response. If there is an obvious improvement, no more medicine may be needed. If there is a slight improvement, repeat doses of the same medicine may be given at approximately 6 or 8 hourly intervals, three or four times. If there is no change at all, a re-assessment and change of medicine or additional help may be needed. For disorders or accidents occurring a few days previously, a useful dosage is more likely to be one tablet three times a day for 2 or 3 days.

Homoeopathic medicines are usually available today as tablets, pillules, drops or as powders suitable for taking by mouth. One tablet, two pillules, two drops, or powder in an amount that would be enough to cover a twenty pence coin usually constitutes one dose. It sometimes surprises people new to homoeopathy to hear that the precise amount given is less critical than the frequency of repetition. We are not so concerned here with material amounts because the medicines are already in a highly reduced form. It has been suggested, for instance, that we would need to take several buckets of belladonna 30C tablets in a short time before a material overdose occurred!

The medicines used in the potentized form are a very fine stimulus dependent more on their quality and timing than their quantity. In this they may be compared to the catalysts studied in chemistry classes. The amount of catalyst added to get a reaction going is less critical than its form.

Another aspect of dosage requirements related to this is that one tablet or drop of medicine is often the required amount for an adult or a child. It is able to offer the stimulus to aid healing whatever the physical weight of the recipient. The timing and quality of the stimulus are more important than whether we give one or two tablets or drops.

Clearly for babies and toddlers drops or powders are easier to take than solid pillules or tablets. If you are using a home first-aid kit that only has tablet preparations, these could be dissolved in a small amount of water or crushed to powder form to make them easier to give to young children. The tablets, powders or pillules all act as carriers for the liquid form of medicine produced by potentization and can be redissolved if this makes dosage easier.

It is often suggested that homoeopathic medicines should be

absorbed from the mouth by sucking tablets slowly or allowing powders to dissolve gradually, and that they should be taken 30 minutes before or after other food or drink. This is a refinement that is not always possible in a first-aid situation. If a toddler has a tumble and produces bruises and grazing some promptly-given *Arnica* is likely to help whether or not he has recently had a meal.

When discussing the use of homoeopathic medicines for first aid it is always important to emphasize that this can be used alongside other appropriate forms of help as required. For any medical need it is important to find adequate help. If a problem looks severe enough from the outset to indicate the need for medical help, the sooner it is requested the better. Even here some appropriate form of homoeopathic medicine may be of assistance while waiting for other help to arrive. For problems that are less severe, like some forms of influenza or minor cuts and bruises that can be safely managed with home first aid, a promptly given homoeopathic medicine can usefully aid the recovery phase to the relief of patients and their families.

The role of homoeopathic medicine as a complementary therapy is as obvious in first aid as it is in many other situations. Good general physical care of patients and their cuts, bruises, more complicated injuries or infections, is clearly important. The use of medicines as a complement to other aspects of therapy and general care is usefully implied when it is described as 'Complementary Medicine'. If necessary homoeopathic medicines can also be used alongside other forms of medication and as an additional aid for patients having surgery. If surgery is imminent and a person has been told not to take anything by mouth then of course oral homoeopathic medicines are also not to be given at that time.

Homoeopathic medicine has often been described as an additional string to the therapeutic bow. When required it can be used in harmony with other forms of therapy. At other times it may be the only form of medicinal stimulus required.

Hahnemann's insights about homoeopathic medicines and how to use them developed steadily through his many years of practice as a physician. The understanding and practice of all forms of medicine, including homoeopathy, has continued advancing since his time. The suggestions contained in this book about ways of using homoeopathic medicine will also probably be modified in due course. The following chapters will, I hope, serve as a guide as home prescribers increase their own use of this form of medicine.

CHAPTER 3

Homoeopathic Aids for the Treatment of Injuries

The aim in this chapter is to consider the various ways in which homoeopathic medicines from the list of twenty can usefully augment the care of a wide range of injuries. General care of an injured person and attention to wounds is obviously important. While appropriate cleansing and dressing of wounds is performed reassurance and practical help can usefully allay anxieties for adults as well as for children.

The additional use of homoeopathic medicines has frequently been found effective in easing many of the physical and emotional symptoms that can occur with injury. We have previously noted the ideal embodied in homoeopathic prescribing of finding a medical stimulus appropriate to psychological as well as physical aspects of the patient's needs. This is applied in first-aid prescribing for injury, when although there is obvious and due attention to the physical results of trauma we can also note other signs of personal distress and take these into account when selecting a medicine.

In hopes of giving information that is easy to read in times of quiet relaxation or study, as well as easy to refer to in an emergency, I will list common injuries alphabetically with comments on medicines previously found useful for such problems. As well as referring to the accidental injuries that commonly occur, we will also consider treatment before and after surgery. It is reasonable to include this here because surgery, although it is planned, controlled and non-accidental, is a type of physical trauma with incisions and after-effects that have many similarities to unexpected injuries.

Bruises

There are two reasons why it is highly appropriate to begin the prescribing data of this short review by referring to the homoeopathic treatment of bruising and the use of *ARNICA*. First, because bruising is probably one of the commonest injuries we experience, occurring with falls, knocks against objects, from pressure effects, accompanying other injuries such as cuts or more serious problems such as fractures. Bruises may be superficial and easily seen, or initially hidden from view and only 'coming out' with superficial signs of discoloration a few days after the injury. Bruising can be very uncomfortable, particularly if it occurs in parts of the body where the associated swelling causes tight pressure effects, so increasing the pain and stiffness. The second reason is that *Arnica* is a particularly widely used homoeopathic medicine and has probably introduced more people to homoeopathy than any other single preparation.

Many examples could be given of the effects of *Arnica*, such as a toddler who fell at home and produced a large bruise on her forehead, a dinghy sailor who banged his shin hard on a thwart (a wooden bar across his boat) and developed a bruise the size of half an egg, or the grandmother who fell off a bicycle causing extensive bruising to her arms. Each of these people had potentized extracts of *Arnica* as tablets soon after the injury and pleasantly surprised themselves and their families by the speed of their recovery. Reports have also come from mountaineers of reducing bruises sustained while climbing by rubbing them with leaves of the plant *Arnica montana* that grows wild in the Alps. Tinctures or creams containing *Arnica* are sometimes still used today, applying them over bruises with intact skin. But as bottles of liquid or tubes of cream are less easy to carry in first-aid kits than are small pots of tablets, and many of us find that the preparations taken orally are at least as effective or more so than local applications, I am going to recommend keeping available such tablets or similar carriers medicated with *Arnica*.

The preparation I advise for first-aid purposes is *Arnica* 30C to be taken, if possible, very soon after an injury. If used in this way I suggest *Arnica* 30C one tablet (or similar dose) at hourly intervals following the injury for three doses and then if the injury is severe enough to need ongoing treatment, one dose again three times the next day or 2-4 days as required. Obviously if an injury is relatively minor treatment may not need continuing beyond the first day, but for longer lasting problems it can be repeated as required. Referring again to the patients already cited as examples, the toddler had her three

Stimulating the body's own defence mechanisms
Arnica 30C – for bruising

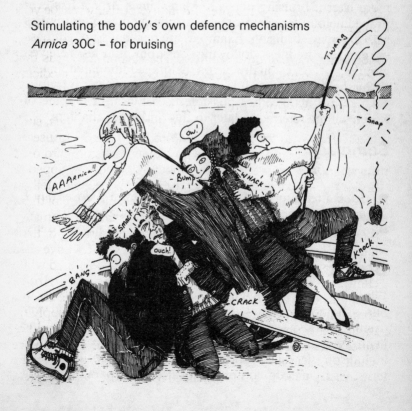

doses of *Arnica* about hourly starting soon after her fall. She settled down generally after a few minutes, and as the bruising was steadily declining after her third dose of *Arnica* was not given any more of it. The dinghy sailor had *Arnica* for 2 days and the grandmother who fell off her bicycle needed it for about 4 days. The duration of the prescription is assessed according to the response. If there has been obvious good relief of symptoms with the shock and bruising markedly better, the doses need not be repeated. If there is a slight improvement it is usually worth continuing the medicine until adequate relief is obtained.

If *Arnica* is not available soon after bruising occurs, it is often worth giving it three times daily for 3–4 days, a week or more later if bruising persists. Many times *Arnica* has ever proved helpful for symptoms occurring months after injuries with extensive bruising. Examples are residual pain, stiffness or general tiredness following on from injuries received months, or occasionally years before additional homoeo-pathic help is requested. Here again, *Arnica* is worth trying.

There are many other possible uses for *Arnica*, some of which will be referred to later in this and other chapters.

Summary

For bruising:

- Soon after injury – *Arnica* 30C hourly for 3–4 doses day 1 followed if required × 3 per day for 3–4 days.
- A few days after injury – *Arnica* 30C × 3 per day 3–4 days.

Burns

While due care is given to the cleansing and dressing of burns, homoeopathic medicines taken by mouth can add very useful general assistance. With small burns pain is often the main general concern; for larger burns the reactions can include physical shock and anxiety as well as pain. The longer term needs include continued local care of painful, oozing burnt surfaces as well as use of medicines that may help reduce more generalized reactions. The homoeopathic medicines appropriate will therefore be considered in three stages: first the acute pain of large or small burns; second, the shock reactions that often accompany burns; and third, the longer term problem of oozing painful wounds.

Acute pain from burns

A homoeopathic medicine particularly useful to relieve pain of burns is *Cantharis*. The use of the medicinal extract of *Cantharis* clearly illustrates the similia principle. The Spanish fly bite can provoke burning pain. An appropriately prepared medicinal extract from this source can treat symptoms that include similar types of pain, particularly the local effects of burns. Many people have found it useful to have a supply of *Cantharis* 30C available in the kitchen as a first-aid measure to ease the discomfort from superficial but painful burns that can easily happen there. If the medicine is being taken very soon after such a burn a useful schedule is one tablet at 30 minute intervals for 3–4 doses as required. As usual with homoeopathic treatment for acute problems, the medicine is stopped as soon as good relief of symptoms occurs.

If homoeopathic medicine is not available for prompt first aid and the pain persists a few days later, it is still worth trying *Cantharis* 30C three times daily for 3–4 days as required.

If burns are extensive and other measures are clearly needed in addition to such simple first aid, *Cantharis* 30C may still help with pain relief.

Shock, or general distress following burns

Such generalized reactions often accompany burns. Large burns with extensive skin loss are physically as well as emotional shocking for patients. Small burns, especially when on particularly sensitive areas such as fingertips can also cause considerable general distress. Adequate treatment of shock and fluid loss, especially likely with extensive burns, is clearly important. Urgent medical help may be needed for this. Even in these circumstances appropriate homoeopathic medicines can be an additional aid to recovery. Two medicines from our group of twenty to consider here are *ACONITE* and *ARNICA*. To decide which to use we will refer to the individual reactions to the trauma as well as the usual effects of burns. The selection process here illustrates the way in which the choice of a homoeopathic medicine even in a first-aid situation can be related to the overall individual reaction as well as particular or localized symptoms.

Aconite 30C is the medicine I would suggest where the shock reaction includes anxiety and restlessness. After burns people are often frightened, agitated and restless. Even if the accident has occurred several minutes or an hour or more previously, a fear reaction accompanied by general restlessness, fidgeting or tears may still be evident. For such reactions we may prescribe *Aconite* 30C at 30 minute intervals for 3–4 doses as required.

Arnica is more likely to help if the individual reaction following injury by burning again includes anxiety but is also accompanied by irritability and withdrawal from people. An example is the person who has obvious pain and some degree of personal shock from a burn but scorns or refuses help. Part of the reaction said to imply the need for homoeopathic *Arnica* is a refusal to accept medical help even though it is clearly needed. Keynotes here to assist the choice of homoeopathic medicines are therefore irritability and anxiety. If the individual can be persuaded to accept it, *Arnica* 30C is likely to be more help here than *Aconite*. Again a useful dosage regimen is *Arnica* 30C at 30-minute intervals for 3–4 doses as required for relief of these immediate effects.

The longer term problem of oozing, painful burnt areas of skin

Suitable dressings or other forms of local wound care are obviously important here. Homoeopathic medicines to be taken by mouth are an additional aid. Such help can come from *KALI BICH*. 30C. This homoeopathic medicine is widely used for medical problems causing sticky discharges and pain in localized areas. Burns can show both of these reactions and the potentized form of *Kali bich*. may therefore be of use in their treatment. A suggested dosage is *Kali bich*. 30C one tablet taken three times daily for 3–4 days until the symptoms improve. It is often helpful to treat the initial shock and acute pain from burns with *Arnica* 30C or *Aconite* 30C, then follow this with *Kali bich*. 30C for the effects that are usually longer lasting.

Summary

For local pain from burns:

- Immediately after the injury – *Cantharis* 30C 1 tablet ½ hourly for 3–4 doses as required.
- A few days later – *Cantharis* 30C 1 tablet 3 times daily for 3–4 days if required.

For shock or general distress:

- With fear and restlessness – *Aconite* 30C 1 table ½ hourly for 3–4 doses as required.
- With fear and irritability – *Arnica* 30C 1 tablet ½ hourly for 3–4 doses as required.

For pain plus continued oozing from burnt skin:

- *Kali bich*. 30C 1 tablet 3 times daily for 3–4 days if required.

Cuts

Three medicines may be considered from the selected twenty here. I will relate them to three particular types of cuts that commonly occur in every-day situations. The three medicines are *ARNICA, STAPHISAGRIA* and *SYMPHYTUM*. The types of cuts for which their use may be considered are:

1. Relatively superficial ones with adjacent bruising or grazes likely to occur when a child falls over.
2. Clean, straight wounds that can easily follow slips with knives or razors.
3. More complicated irregular injuries with underlying problems as well as surface cuts such as occur with heavy falls or road accidents.

For all of these, careful cleansing and dressings are required. If internal injuries are suspected it is important to get medical help as soon as possible. This is similarly required if cuts to fingers or wrists are thought to have damaged underlying nerves, muscles or tendons controlling the sensations and movements of the hands. Even when such help is being sought appropriate homoeopathic medicines may be used for additional aid.

Simple cuts with bruising

A common occurrence for people of all ages. Whether the injury affects a stumbling toddler, a DIY enthusiast who misdirects his hammer, or an elderly person who falls, the resulting superficial but unpleasant cuts and bruises can often be quickly helped by *Arnica*. It is more effective if given soon after an injury. A useful dosage is *Arnica* 30C one tablet at 30 minute intervals; often two or three doses are sufficient.

Clean, straight cuts

Sharp and clean kitchen knives can easily slip and cause such injuries which, even if they are relatively superficial, can bleed easily and be very uncomfortable. Pain can be a particular problem when fingers are injured because of the large number of nerve endings there to increase sensitivity. A homoeopathic medicine indicated here is *Staphisagria*. Used soon after straight clean cuts, it can often quickly help to reduce pain and bleeding. A suggested dosage is *Staphisagria* 30C one tablet at 30 minute intervals. Three to four doses are usually sufficient.

Deep cuts, irregular with additional injuries

Examples of the type of injury considered here are the effects of road accidents, where additional medical help is needed and homoeopathic medicines are given as additional first aid. *Arnica* may be useful as a starter, particularly if the patient is shocked as well as physically injured. Provided the patient can safely have medicines by mouth, one tablet at 30 minute intervals for 3 doses is again often appropriate.

Following on from this, another useful homoeopathic prescription is *Symphytum*. In its potentized form this medicine has been found an effective aid to the healing of complicated soft-tissue injuries. It has also been widely used to assist healing of fractures, an application we will emphasize later in this chapter. It is therefore a particularly useful homoeopathic medicine for complex injuries affecting soft tissues as well as bones. Like other homoeopathic medicines it can be given in conjunction with treatment of a non-homoeopathic form also likely to be required for complicated injuries. A suggested dosage is *Symphytum* 30C one tablet three times daily for 3 days after the course of arnica. When extensive injuries need treatment over several weeks it may also be useful to repeat the prescription of *Symphytum* 30C three times a day for one day each week.

Summary

For simple cuts and grazes with bruising:

- Soon after injury – *Arnica* 30C 1 tablet ½ hourly for 2–3 doses.

For straight clean cuts:

- Soon after injury – *Staphisagria* 30C 1 tablet ½ hourly for 3–4 doses.

For severe complicated cuts:

- For shock soon after injury *Arnica* 30C 1 tablet ½ hourly 3 doses followed by *Symphytum* 30C 1 tablet 3 times daily for 3 days followed if needed by 1 tablet 3 times daily 1 day per week.

Eye injuries

The sort of injuries considered here can easily occur when someone is hit close to or over the eye with bruising and perhaps cuts around it and also possible redness of the eyeball. These injuries are often particularly difficult to assess. If they are obviously superficial injuries of eyelids, basic first aid may be all that is required. But if there is any suspicion that the eye itself is affected it is important to seek expert assessment as soon as possible. Appropriate homoeopathic medicines may be given while waiting for such help. Three relevant homoeopathic medicines are *ARNICA, LEDUM* and *SYMPHYTUM*. Sometimes it can be difficult to decide which one is most likely to help an individual. As basic first aid that can be used at home is being considered, I suggest a simple assessment based on the type of pain and some other obvious features about the injury and its effects. It is an example of the way in which the quality of pain can be one of the factors that can help determine which homoeopathic medicine to use.

Non-severe bruising and soreness

The sort of injury that may follow falls causing grazing around the eye and eyelids with soreness and aching. Here I suggest *Arnica* 30C one tablet hourly for 3–4 doses as required.

More severe injuries with obvious blackness around the eye and redness of the eyeball

For complex injuries of this sort it is advisable to have expert assessment. While waiting for that, a single dose of *Arnica* 30C is a useful aid for treating the general shock reaction and pain that commonly accompanies severe eye injuries. Following this, about 20 minutes later, I suggest *Ledum* 30C repeated hourly for three doses and also three times on the following day.

Persisting pain following eye injuries

Where pain is particularly severe or continues despite appropriate treatment and *Arnica* or *Ledum*, I suggest *Symphytum* 30C with one dose three times a day for 3 days if required.

Summary

Non-severe bruising and soreness:

* *Arnica* 30C 1 tablet hourly × 3–4.

Severe injury, obvious discoloration and shock:

* *Arnica* 30C 1 tablet followed by *Ledum* 30C 1 hourly × 3 and 1 tablet 3 times the next day.

Persisting pain from eye injury:

* *Symphytum* 30C 1 tablet × 3 daily for 3 days if required.

Fractures

A fracture of a bone should be considered if following injury to it there is severe pain, general shock or obvious alteration in shape. In these circumstances medical assessment is needed. Homoeopathic medicines can augment both the first aid offered and the on-going care of fractures. We will look first at homoeopathic treatment for shock accompanying fractures and secondly at medicines to help with the more localized healing of the fracture site.

Shock accompanying fractures

Most fractures are likely to be accompanied by an initial general distress. The patient may feel breathless, faint, cold or anxious as well as having a fast heartbeat and perhaps showing a tendency to faint. Such reactions can be a sign of individual shock that may well accompany injury severe enough to cause a bone fracture. A medicine indicated here is *Arnica* 30C with one dose at 30 minute intervals for 2–3 doses if required. Many reports have been given of the beneficial effects of this medicine in such a situation with prompt relief of many of the general effects of the injury.

To assist healing at a fracture site

Two medicines from the selected twenty to consider here are *Arnica* and *Symphytum*. *Arnica* 30C is particularly useful for helping to reduce soft-tissue injury such as bruising and swelling around fracture sites, *Symphytum* 30C is more suited to assisting healing of bone. They therefore usefully complement each other in fracture care. For a dosage regimen I suggest *Arnica* 30C three times a day for 3 days followed by *Symphytum* 30C twice daily for 1 week.

Summary

For shock following a fracture:

- *Arnica* 30C 1 tablet ½ hourly × 2–3.

For bruising at fracture site:

- *Arnica* 30C 1 tablet 3 times daily for 3 days.

To assist bone repair:

- *Symphytum* 30C 1 tablet twice daily for 1 week.

Insect bites

One way of choosing a homoeopathic medicine to ease the effects of such injuries is to consider the particular features of the reaction provoked. Common effects of any insect bite can be redness, some degree of swelling at the site and pain that may be a general soreness or more of an irritation. Such reactions are due to the chemical stimulus of the bite and the individual reaction of the person experiencing it. The particular type of reaction evoked can guide us to a homoeopathic medicine likely to reduce it. Two medicines from our twenty to consider here are *CANTHARIS* and *LEDUM*.

Ledum 30C – for insect bites

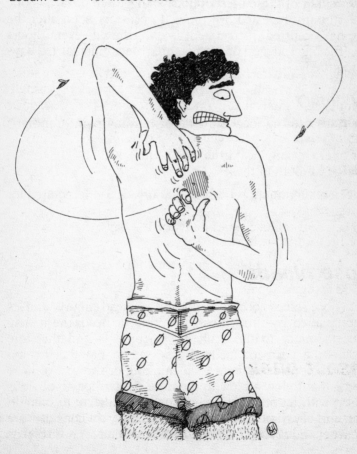

As we noted previously when looking at medicines for burns, *Cantharis* 30C is particularly indicated for the relief of pain that has a burning or stinging quality. It is therefore an appropriate medicine for bites when the local redness and swelling are associated with this type of discomfort.

Ledum 30C is appropriate when the pain is more irritant in quality so that there is an urge to scratch the site. A keynote about the irritation suggesting a need for *Ledum* is that scratching intensifies rather than relieves it.

For either of these prescriptions a suggested dosage is one tablet hourly repeated 3–4 times if necessary soon after the bite has occurred. If treatment is only started several hours after the bite I suggest one tablet three times daily for 1–2 days as required.

Summary

For bites causing local stinging or burning pain: *Cantharis* 30C.

For bites causing local irritation: *Ledum* 30C.

Dosage for both of these:

- Soon after injury – 1 tablet ½ hourly × 3–4 if required for relief.
- Later – 1 tablet 3 times daily for 1–2 days.

Nose bleeds

If a nose bleed occurs following a head injury and is accompanied by drowsiness, vomiting or headache it may indicate injury to the skull or its contents and therefore implies the need for medical assessment. For the first-aid purposes considered here I am thinking or the sort of nose bleeds that follow a blow to the nose or start for no obvious reason with no major injury suspected. They are a common problem. Two of our twenty medicines to consider are *ARNICA* and *PHOSPHORUS*. Both are useful for nose bleeds

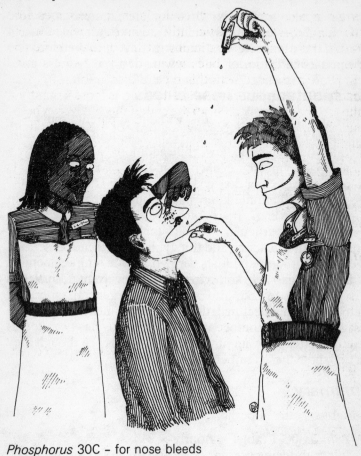

Phosphorus 30C – for nose bleeds

and if only one of them is available it is usually worthwhile using it. If both are available, we can select one or the other by noting the likely cause of the nose bleed and its particular characteristics.

For nose bleeds after superficial injury

A blow to the nose with damage to superficial blood vessels may result in slight or sometimes heavy local blood loss.

There may also be adjacent bruising. Here a useful medicine is *Arnica* 30C with one dose at 30 minute intervals for 3-4 doses. If there is severe local bruising the *Arnica* could also be repeated for three doses the following day.

For spontaneous nose bleeds

When the nose bleed occurs without apparent injury – a common example is with colds – gentle but firm local pressure will often help stem the flow while additional aid is given by a homoeopathic medicine taken by mouth. *Phosphorus* 30C is often useful here. For dosage I suggest using *Phosphorus* 30C one tablet at 30 minute intervals 3-4 times if required to help stop the bleeding. It is often said that homoeopathic *Phosphorus* is particularly helpful for people who are chilly, sensitive, quick reacting and thirsty. It is sometimes described briefly as suiting individuals with an artistic temperament. If we are seeking to help someone who has recurrent nose bleeds it is important to take into account such general aspects of their profile in selecting a homoeopathic medicine. But for first-aid purposes homoeopathic *Phosphorus* has been found helpful for treating patients with nose bleeds even though they do not show these temperamental features.

Summary

Nose bleed after superficial injury:

- *Arnica* 30C 1 tablet ½ hourly × 3-4.
- If local bruising present – repeat *Arnica* 30C × 3 next day.

Spontaneous nose bleed – *Phosphorus* 30C 1 tablet ½ hourly × 3-4.

Puncture wounds

Here we may consider injuries such as needle jabs while sewing, stab type wounds from slips with kitchen knives as well as the effects of people of any age falling onto sharp points. Another cause may be a dog bite. Local cleaning of the wound can be accompanied by the use of homoeopathic medicine to ease the discomfort. The type of pain can again be used as a guide in selecting a particular medicine. A throbbing or pricking quality to the pain, which is uncomfortable but not severe, is a pointer to using *LEDUM*. Where the pain from a puncture wound is severe an appropriate homoeopathic medicine is more likely to be *STAPHISAGRIA*. Either of these can be used in the 30C potency with one dose repeated at 30-minute intervals for 3–4 doses if required for relief of pain.

Summary

Puncture wounds with pricking or throbbing discomfort:

● *Ledum* 30C.
Puncture wounds with marked pain:
● *Staphisagria* 30C.
Dosage for either of these – 1 tablet ½ hourly × 3–4 if required.

Sprains

While appropriate local dressings or strappings may be required to support the sprained ligaments or tendons, further help can be obtained by taking homoeopathic medicines by mouth. Two that have often been useful for this type of injury are *ARNICA* and *RHUS TOX*. For sprains occurring in adults or children both of these medicines are likely to help reduce the pain and swelling. I have found it better to use *Arnica* first soon after the injury particularly when there is bruising of the area and pain on moving the joint. If the medicine is being given immediately after the injury I suggest *Arnica* 30C hourly for four doses, and repeated three times the following day if severe bruising has occurred.

When the acute pain and bruising has eased and the joint shows residual stiffness that can be eased by gentle movement, *Rhus tox.* 30C is more likely to be helpful. For dosage I suggest one tablet given three times daily for 3–4 days as required for relief.

Summary

Soon after sprain, for bruising and pain:

● *Arnica* 30C 1 tablet ½ hourly × 4.

Later, if required for stiffness:

● *Rhus tox.* 30C 1 tablet × 3 daily 3–4 days.

Pre- and post-operation

For first-aid purposes there are two medicines in the twenty that have often been found useful for extra help when given alongside the conventional treatment offered before and after surgery. These are *ARNICA* and *STAPHISAGRIA*. For both of these medicines we are considering a specific application of the indications we noted for their use earlier in this chapter. That is, *Arnica* to help reduce bruising and *Staphisagria* to reduce pain and assist healing of clean, incised wounds.

Arnica 30C has been widely used to assist by reducing bruising, which eases post-operative discomfort and facilitates healing. Most operations are likely to incur bruising to some degree. When *Arnica* 30C can help reduce this it can be an extra aid to recovery. For surgical procedures as diverse as tonsillectomy, hip replacement or appendicectomy, *Arnica* can be an additional aid. A regimen for dosage often found useful is *Arnica* 30C one tablet the day before surgery, for instance the evening before an operation due the following morning. And *Arnica* 30C three times daily for 3 or 4 days post-operatively.

If pain is particularly severe following surgery additional help may also be obtained from *Staphisagria* 30C one tablet taken three times daily if required for 6–7 days. As usual with homoeopathic medicines, these preparations can be used alongside other treatment.

Summary

To help reduce bruising and so assist pain control and healing:

- *Arnica* 30C: The day before surgery – 1 tablet.
                    Following surgery – 1 tablet
                    × 3 daily 3–4 days.

For additional help with severe pain after an operation:

- *Staphisagria* 30C 1 tablet × 3 daily 6–7 days as needed.

CHAPTER 4

Homoeopathic Aids for Common Problems of Children

The type of problems considered here are first infectious diseases that children often develop, second some of the sleep problems that frequently occur and in the third section a few other common difficulties such as teething and temper tantrums. They are all problems which, though unlikely to be medically serious, can be very distressing for the children concerned and their families and where homoeopathic first aid can often be usefully applied. We know that infectious problems such as chicken-pox and mumps are usually gradually overcome without lasting damage; but even so their course can be very unpleasant for all concerned, and if a homoeopathic medicine can relieve the effects and hasten recovery this is obviously useful.

We will see in discussing the selection of homoeopathic medicines that may help such difficulties how we need to take note of an individual patient's general reactions occurring with a disease as well as the more localized symptoms. In the previous chapter when we were looking at ways of helping acute injuries of various forms, there was an emphasis on noting the particular effects of the trauma in order to select a homoeopathic medicine. In this chapter more stress is placed on taking a holistic review of the patient's profile. That includes noting an individual patient's general reactions to the disease as well as its more localized effects. An example would be prescribing for a child with a cold after noting changes in his general behaviour as well as his eyes, nose and throat symptoms. It illustrates the aim discussed in the first chapter of finding a medicine to suit the overall profile of the person seeking help.

Infectious diseases

Chicken-pox

A common and unpleasant disease, but fortunately one where major complications are rare and homoeopathic medicines can usefully augment the general care of the patients and their skin lesions. Occasionally chicken-pox can lead on to more serious forms of infection in the spots or to other general disorders. If a child is acutely ill or his skin lesions are obviously infected, it is advisable to seek additional medical help. With the commoner less complicated but still unpleasant forms of chicken-pox, homoeopathic medicines may be the main medical aid.

The spots tend to come up in groups; they can occur on most parts of the body but are particularly seen on the trunk. They progress from a small red area, to more obvious spots with a vesicle that gradually dries and crusts. It is a counsel of perfection to advise not scratching(!) but it reduces the risks of infection. If homoeopathic medicines can be started early in the infection, their benefit is usually greater.

The medicines from our present kit to consider here are *ANTIMONIUM TARTRATE, PULSATILLA* and *RHUS TOX*. The guides to assist a decision on which of these three to select can be found in the general demeanour of the patient.

Antimonium tartrate 30C is indicated where a child is peevish and despondent with the disease. Typically children needing *Ant. tart.* are moody, fed up and difficult to cheer up. They tend to whine and shy away from touch.

Children for whom *Pulsatilla* 30C is more likly to help may also be prone to whining and moodiness. But a marked difference here is in the response to touch and affection.

Children needing *Pulsatilla* welcome affection. They want to be held. Other features that suggest *Pulsatilla* as a suitable medicine are dislike of hot rooms, tearfulness and lack of thirst.

The third medicine, *Rhus tox.* 30C, can be selected according to the degree of restlessness. It is more likely to suit children who show their agitation with their irritating spots by tossing around or refusing to stay in bed. Often there is a marked mood change with either anxiety of dejection notably different from the norm for the individual patient.

Looking at the children for their general reactions in this way can help to decide which medicine to advise. They may all show similar skin changes, but the individual reactions accompanying them vary greatly and can indicate the medicine likely to give more help. For all three I suggest using the medicine in the 30C potency, with one dose four times daily while the child is ill enough to need it.

Summary

For chicken-pox:

- In a peevish child opposing being held – *Ant. tart.* 30C.
- In a whining child craving attention – *Pulsatilla* 30C.
- In a very restless, irritable child – *Rhus tox.* 30C.

Dosage for all three – 1 tablet × 4 per day up to 5 days.

Ear infections

Homoeopathic medicines can be used in the treatment of ear infections either as first aid for early symptoms when hopefully the medicine may avert the need for something stronger, or as an addition to prescriptions of a more conventional nature if established infection is already being treated. In either of these situations suitable homoeopathic treatment can give useful benefit.

One way of choosing which homoeopathic medicine to use is to consider them in two groups. The first refers to medicines indicated for ear infections causing pain without discharge.

The second is for infections where both of these effects are evident. When prescribing for children with ear infections in either of these categories we need to note their general reactions and behaviour as well as the details concerning the symptoms focused on the ear. There may also be a need for medical advice. For ear pain without discharge this should be sought if symptoms do not improve within 6 hours. When an ear discharges, with or without pain, a doctor's examination and advice are needed from the start with the homoeopathic medicines used as an additional aid.

Ear pain from early infection with no discharge

Two medicines from our selected twenty to consider here are *ACONITE* and *BELLADONNA*. Since both can be appropriate for early stages of infection with pain, restlessness and slightly raised temperature, it can be difficult to decide on which of them to use. Details of the type of pain as well as the general reactions can help us select one.

The type of pain particularly likely to be helped by *Aconite* 30C is described as stitching, tearing or pricking. The individual reaction accompanying it includes irritability and anxiety as well as restlessness.

When *Belladonna* 30C is more likely to help, the ear pain is more of a burning and throbbing character and the general reaction to it marked agitation or irritability in the child with marked restlessness. Another small point that can help us decide which medicine to use is the size of the pupils which tend to be widely dilated when homoeopathic *Belladonna* is likely to be useful.

With both medicines a suggested prescription for use early in the development of the symptoms is one tablet of the 30C potency repeated hourly 3–4 times if required.

Ear pain from infection with discharge

Three medicines to consider here are potentized extracts of *KALI BICH.*, *MERC. SOL.* and *PULSATILLA*. The particular form of the discharge from the ear as well as the overall state of the patient need taking into account to help select one of these for use. Medical advice is also important here as other forms of treatment may be required for individuals with such problems.

A need for *Kali bich.* 30C is indicated by a thick, stringy and yellowish discharge. This medicine is useful for many catarrhal or discharging conditions and a recurrent feature is the stringy character of the exudate. The general reaction includes a tendency to listless irritability and tiredness, like a child who complains he is bored but cannot settle himself to try to do something.

With the problems more likely to be helped by *Merc. sol.* 30C again there is tiredness and irritability but here there is also marked restlessness. The child who needs this medicine may be prone to wander around or fidget recurrently and show a generally anxious temperament. The discharge from the ear is offensive and messy, and the ear is generally sore or tender. These features all suggest the need for potentized *Merc. sol.*

The third medicine we can consider here is *Pulsatilla* 30C. This is indicated where the discharge is again thick and yellowish but its character is much more bland or smooth. The child who needs this medicine is generally sensitive, moody, clinging to its parents and showing very little thirst.

For dosage with any of these three medicines for children with discharging infected ears, I suggest one tablet or two drops if these are easier to give, of the 30C potency repeated three times daily for 3-4 days as required. They can all be used as an additional aid to other forms of medical help as required.

Summary

For early stages of ear infection, with pain and no discharge:

- Sharp pains in a slightly restless child - *Aconite* 30C.
- Throbbing, burning pain in a very restless child - *Belladonna* 30C.
- Dosage - 1 tablet hourly for 3-4 times.

For ear infection with discharge:

- Stringy, yellow discharge with a listless tired child – *Kali bich*. 30C.
- Messy, offensive discharge with a restless irritable child – *Merc. sol*. 30C.
- Bland yellow discharge in a whining, clinging child – *Pulsatilla* 30C.
- Dosage – 1 tablet or its equivalent × 3 per day, 3–4 days if required.

Measles

When this common infection occurs without complications homoeopathic medicines can often ease its severity sufficiently to avert the need for stronger forms of treatment. We need, however, to be wary of ear infections developing with it. Other complications are very rare, but if a child is showing signs of persisting ear problems or more serious general disease, it is wise to ask for a medical check. Even uncomplicated measles can be very unpleasant with its general debility, sore eyes, irritating cough and skin eruption, so any help given with homoeopathic medicines can be a relief to the parents as well as to the child.

From our twenty medicines I suggest *ARSENICUM ALBUM, BELLADONNA, KALI BICH*. and *PULSATILLA*. The selection of just one of these will depend on which measles symptoms are particularly prominent as well as the general reaction of the child.

Arsenicum album 30C is useful when the eyes and throat are sore and burning, the cough as if from a dry tickle in the throat and the skin showing the typical measles rash. Although homoeopathic *Arsenicum* suits problems where there is burning discomfort, the general reaction includes being chilly and perhaps shivering. The profile here characteristically presents the combination of local burning pains but overall coldness. The general appearance also includes a marked degree of anxious restlessness.

When *Belladonna* 30C is more likely to help the child with measles, the profile again shows the usual effects of the disease but the eyes and lips look particularly red, the skin eruption is florid but with pallor around the mouth, and the pupils may appear dilated. The general reaction includes marked restlessness with the temperature and cough.

Kali bich. 30C is indicated if the child is excessively catarrhal with his or her measles, with a loose, thick-sounding cough and marked watering of the eyes. The general reaction suggesting *Kali bich.* as a prescription is tiredness, weariness or apathy.

Pulsatilla 30C – for measles

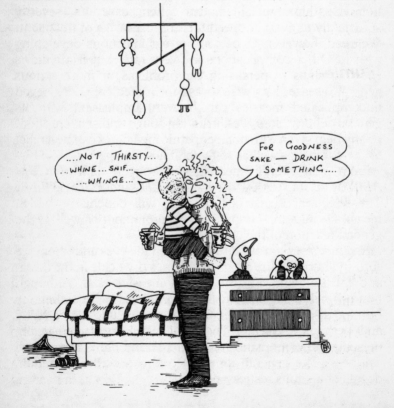

When *Pulsatilla* 30C is more likely to help, the measles symptoms are again accompanied by marked watering of the eyes and a loose or tickle type of cough but the general reaction includes whining, craving of attention, tearfulness and lack of thirst.

Sometimes it is useful to follow on from one medicine to another. For instance, we may need to give *Pulsatilla* as the measles begins with eye symptoms, a tickly cough in a child generally unwell and craving attention. If this is followed by symptoms with a change to stringy catarrh, we may follow on with *Kali bich*. Or if heat and restlessness are prevalent at one stage, and burning eyes and fidgety agitation at another time, *Belladonna* may be needed first, *Arsenicum album* later. For dosage I suggest the 30C potency of these medicines, used 2 hourly if symptoms are of recent onset for 3-4 doses if required.

Summary

Measles:

- With burning discomfort in a chilly restless child – *Ars. alb*. 30C.
- With florid red skin rash, eyes and lips in a chilly, cross, very restless child – *Belladonna* 30C.
- With a lot of catarrh in a tired listless child – *Kali bich*. 30C.
- In a clinging, whining, tearful, thirstless child – *Pulsatilla*. 30C.
- Dosage for all of these: 1 tablet 2 hourly × 3-4 if required.

Mumps

For the pain and swelling of the parotid gland that commonly accompany mumps we can consider using *BELLADONNA, CHAMOMILLA* and *MERC. SOL*. Such local changes are sometimes the first obvious sign of the infection. Alternatively there may also be a short period of general ill health and a raised temperature before the obvious changes in the parotid gland which are the hallmark of mumps. The localized pain in this gland can be quite severe, especially when eating, so a homoeopathic medicine that may reduce it can be very welcome.

Belladonna 30C is indicated when the appearance of the child appears red and hot. The child looks flushed, is very restless and has sudden surges of burning or throbbing pain in the inflamed gland.

Chamomilla 30C is indicated when the child is particularly irritable or even angry with the mumps infection and tends to reject the attention and care offered. The pain is often in paroxysms, stitching or burning in character.

When the pain is more of a tearing character we should consider using *Merc. sol*. 30C. As usual for mumps the pain is worse on attempting to eat or even sometimes on talking. But if it is tearing or drawing in quality this can be a guide to using *Merc. sol*. Other local features that also suggest using this medicine are profuse salivation and indentation along the tongue as if it were soft and has been pushed onto the teeth. The more general features include restlessness, irritability and a tendency to be despondent.

I suggest using the 30C potency of any of these medicines three times daily for 3–4 days if required.

Summary

For mumps:

- In a flushed, restless child with burning pain – *Belladonna* 30C.
- In an irritable, angry child with stitching or burning pain – *Chamomilla* 30C.
- In a despondent, restless child with heavy salivation – *Merc. sol*. 30C.
- Dosage – 1 tablet × 3 daily 3–4 days as required.

Tonsillitis

Another common problem in children and adults, and one

where prompt use of a homoeopathic medicine may reduce or avert the need for stronger prescriptions. I shall look particularly at the use of *ACONITE, BELLADONNA, CANTHARIS* and *MERC. SOL*.

The indications for using *Aconite* 30C include inflammation of the throat with scraping, pressing or stitching discomfort there. It provokes an inclination to swallow but this aggravates

Belladonna 30C – for tonsillitis

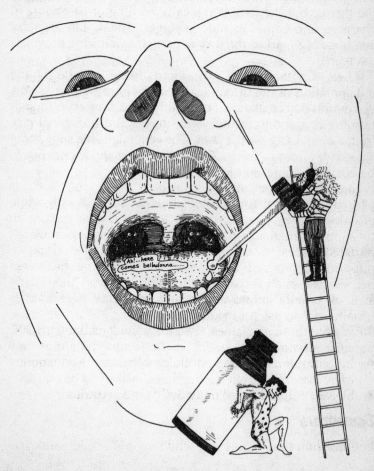

the discomfort. The general reaction accompanying it includes anxious restlessness and irritability, especially at night. Overheating or coldness can make the patient feel worse.

With the symptom picture suggesting a need for *Belladonna* 30C there is again irritability and restlessness but to an even greater degree than in a patient needing *Aconite*. The appearance in the *Belladonna* profile again includes redness and heat in reaction to the temperature and marked redness of the throat, but the pain is typically burning or throbbing in character and comes in sudden surges. The mouth feels dry and there is a marked thirst even though swallowing provokes the pain.

When *Cantharis* 30C is more likely to help, the inflammation of the throat again causes burning pains. This discomfort is accentuated if the child has cold water. Although burning is a strong feature here, local warmth, for instance from a scarf, can ease the pain. The general profile suggesting a need for *Cantharis* includes anxiety, anger and a tendency to be busy but achieve little.

The fourth medicine to consider, *Merc. sol.* 30C, is particularly useful for the tonsillitis associated with white discoloration in patches on the tonsils. If this is seen in tonsillitis, particularly in a despondent, restless person who is prone to profuse sweating and salivation, it is often useful to prescribe potentized *Merc. sol.* This medicine has often helped clear such throat infections. If, however, there is no sign of prompt improvement and problems persist, it is usually wise to ask for medical help.

For all of these medicines, used for acute tonsillitis, the 30C potency may be given hourly if the symptoms are of very recent onset, for 3–4 doses. If the problem has been niggling for a few days a more effective regimen is likely to be one dose of the 30C potency three times daily for 3–4 days.

Summary

For tonsillitis:

- In a restless anxious child with scraping throat pain – *Aconite* 30C.
- In a very restless flushed child with burning and throbbing throat pain – *Belladonna* 30C.
- In an angry child with burning pain eased by keeping warm – *Cantharis* 30C.
- In a restless child with white exudate on the tonsils – *Merc. sol.* 30C.
- Dosage:
  For very recent symptoms – 1 dose hourly × 3–4 if required.
  For longer lasting symptoms – 1 dose × 3 per day for 3–4 days if required.

Sleep problems

Insomnia (sleeplessness)

The emphasis in homoeopathic medicine on assessing the causes of symptoms and taking these into account when advising treatment is clearly illustrated in seeking to help children, or adults, suffering from sleeplessness. To select a prescription we need to consider the likely provoking factors and the temperament of the child reacting to them as well as the particular type of sleep disturbance that is shown. With this aim in mind I therefore suggest selecting first-aid remedies according to the circumstances in which the sleeplessness occurs and the child's general state.

Anxiety-provoking situations

It is usually relatively easy to spot tension or anxiety prior to examinations, special events at school or moves between classes. It is often less easy to notice children reacting to pressures at home or from their friends and to assess the effect this is having in provoking anxiety and disrupting their sleep. Where such pressures can be identified it is clearly better if the problems can be discussed and perhaps modified. If, despite such measures, sleeplessness remains a difficulty, two of the twenty homoeopathic medicines are particularly worth considering for use.

For a chilly, restless, tidy and generally tense child we may advise *ARSENICUM ALBUM* 30C.

For a child who looks hot but may complain of feeling cold, is very restless, recurrently wakes up feeling frightened and perhaps has frightening dreams, *BELLADONNA* 30C is more likely to be helpful.

Overtiredness leading to sleeplessness

A common problem and one for which there are two medicines in the list to consider.

In a child who is easily apprehensive in many circumstances so has been over-excited by even minor exertions, *ARSENICUM ALBUM* 30C is suggested.

For a child who is usually not easily over-stimulated and can usually cope with his routine I have found *ARNICA* 30C helpful.

Difficulty sleeping after over-eating

The homoeopathic medicine likely to help here is *NUX VOMICA* 30. It is particularly useful for the irritable restlessness that can occur if children have become over-excited as well as overfed at parties.

Sleeping problems with homesickness

For children showing this problem I suggest *ARSENICUM ALBUM* or *PULSATILLA*.

Arsenicum album 30C, as noted before, is indicated for a restless, generally tense, chilly, organized child.

Pulsatilla 30C is more likely to help the child who is yielding, placid and inclined to cling and whine.

Two other common factors in sleeplessness in children are colic and teething. Homoeopathic help for these difficulties will be considered later in this chapter.

Summary

Sleeplessness:

- From anxiety – *Ars. alb.* 30C or *Belladonna* 30C.
- In over-tired children – *Ars. alb.* 30C or *Arnica* 30C.
- After over-eating – *Nux. vom.* 30C.
- With homesickness – *Pulsatilla* 30C.
- Dosage for all of these – 1 tablet at night if required.

Nightmares

Another common problem where the use of a homoeopathic medicine may help settle not only the frightened child but therefore indirectly the parents. Three of our twenty selected homoeopathic medicines warrant particular consideration here and again the general temperament of the child can be the guide to choosing just one of them for use. The three medicines to look at are *Ant. tart.*, *Arsenicum album*, and *Pulsatilla*. All three can be suitable for the child showing the familiar reaction of waking up very frightened after nightmares.

Ant. tart. 30C is particularly suitable for a child who is often peevish, easily gets cross, tends to whine and resists being picked up.

The general profile for a child where *Arsenicum album* 30C is more likely to help includes a tendency to be fastidious, easily anxious in the day as well as night, chilly and prone to fidget. They are particularly prone to wake feeling anxious and restless shortly after midnight.

When *Pulsatilla* 30C is indicated the temperament is more easy going, a child who gives way easily, tends to moods or perhaps to be sulky, craves attention and is generally intolerant of stuffy heat.

Summary

Nightmares:

- In a child prone to be peevish and cross – *Ant. tart* 30C.

- In a child prone to be fussy, restless and anxious – *Ars. alb*. 30C.
- In a child prone to be gentle, yielding but moody – *Pulsatilla* 30C.
- Dosage for any of these – 1 tablet at night if required.

Sleep-walking

Although this problem is usually less common than nightmares in children, it occurs often enough to lead to its inclusion in this short book. Two medicines to consider for a child prone to sleep-walking are *ACONITE* and *NATRUM MUR*.

Aconite 30C is more likely to help when the sleep-walking seems to be a continuation of anxieties often shown in the day as well as night. A general state of agitation, being easily upset and fearful, with restlessness and dislike of both cold and heat, is a guide to a need for *Aconite*.

The other medicine to consider here, *Natrum mur*. 30C, is better suited to the child who generally is not obviously anxious but develops sleep problems and sleep-walking after a particular fright or major upset. It is particularly useful for children reacting to bereavements in the family, or the loss of much loved pets. Even if the emotional reaction to this type of loss is not obvious, if sleep disturbance develops coincident with it, *Natrum mur*. 30C may usefully help.

Summary

Sleep-walking:

- In a generally anxious child – *Aconite* 30C.
- In a child after shock or major loss – *Natrum mur* 30C.
- Dosage for both of these – 1 tablet at night as required.

Other common problems

Teething

Homoeopathic medicines have often proved useful for many

of the reactions shown by children while teething. For restlessness, sleep upsets, local soreness and the various mood changes frequently seen in children at this time two medicines to consider are *CHAMOMILLA* and *PULSATILLA*. The particular details of the mood changes with the teething process can help us decide which to use.

When the child concerned is fractious, irritable, fretful and resists attention, it suggests the need for *Chamomilla* 30C. If a child who usually accepts affection becomes so irritable when teething that he rejects such care, this is a keynote indication for a prescription of *Chamomilla* 30C.

If in contrast to this there is less anger in the reaction and more of a tendency to whine and cling to helpers, the indicated medicine is more likely to be *Pulsatilla* 30C. A

Chamomilla 30C – for teething

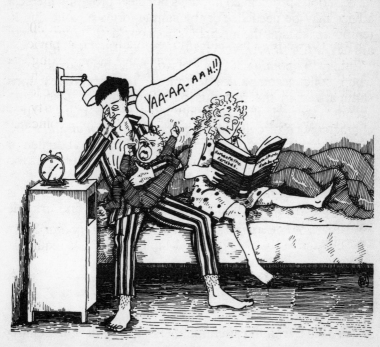

moody, simmering discontent, or tears with requests for attention, are the hallmarks indicating a need for *Pulsatilla*.

Summary

Teething problems:

- In an irritable child rejecting attention – *Chamomilla* 30C.
- In a moody child seeking attention – *Pulsatilla* 30C.
- Dosage for both of these – 1 tablet as required.

Colic

The suggestions here concern the short sharp colic that occurs in a generally healthy baby. Frequently this is associated with a brief episode of spasm that homoeopathic medicine can often usefully relieve. Occasionally, colic may be sign of a more serious problem so if it does not clear promptly medical advice may be needed. For the simple forms of colic due to temporary spasms the medicines from our kit to be considered are *CHAMOMILLA, NUX VOMICA*, and *PULSATILLA*.

Either *Chamomilla* 30C or *Pulsatilla* 30C may be indicated when colic accompanies teething. The general reactions summarized in the previous paragraph can be taken into account to aid the selection of one of them. Other characteristics of colic likely to be eased by *Pulsatilla* 30C include that it is eased by gentle pressure on the abdomen or by bending forwards, but becomes worse if the child gets too hot.

The third medicine to look at here, *Nux vomica* 30C is suggested when the child is generally fractious and irritable with colic that is eased by local warmth but is worse for pressure.

Summary

Colic:

- In a teething, fractious child – *Chamomilla* 30C.
- In a child wanting attention, bending double and seeming

worse for warmth - *Pulsatilla* 30C.
- In an irritable child with colic eased by warmth but worse for pressure - *Nux vom*. 30C.
- Dosage - 1 tablet when required.

Temper tantrums

Here we may think of using potentized *BELLADONNA* and *CHAMOMILLA*. Both can be helpful for children showing outbursts of temper with shouting, throwing things around or even trying to bite helpers. To distinguish which to select we can take into account the general appearance and physical reactions of the child.

Belladonna 30C is more likely to help a child who looks flushed or perhaps even appears hot so that his body as well as his temper looks fiery. The rages come on very suddenly in children where *Belladonna* is indicated. Another marked feature here is anxiety; the child looks frightened as well as angry.

The child who needs *Chamomilla* 30C may also seem worse for becoming heated, but generally has a less florid appearance. His demeanour is generally irritable and impatient instead of frightened and anxious as commonly occurs when *Belladonna* is needed.

Summary

Temper tantrums:

- Occurring very suddenly, in child who looks flushed and frightened - *Belladonna* 30C.
- Occurring in a generally irritable but less anxious child - *Chamomilla* 30C.
- Dosage - 1 tablet as required.

Hay fever

If hay fever symptoms are severe and recurrent they are likely to need assessing in more detail than is covered by the summaries in this review. Here I am thinking of hay fever episodes newly or occasionally occurring where first aid may be requested. For this we may consider *ARSENICUM ALBUM, NUX VOMICA* and *PULSATILLA.*

A need for *Arsenicum album* 30C is suggested by redness of the eyes and nose associated with a corrosive, burning type of discharge. There may be a tendency to wheeze, especially around midnight, and generally the child is restless, fussy, chilly and anxious.

Nux vomica 30C is also indicated for a chilly, fussy child; but here, although the eyes and nose show a lot of watery discharge, this is less corrosive. Irritation of the nose is likely to be marked when homoeopathic *Nux vomica* is indicated.

The need for *Pulsatilla* 30C is also suggested by a profuse watery discharge from the nose and eyes but here it is bland. The general features are also very different when *Pulsatilla* is indicated. Here the child is usually easy going, sensitive, moody and intolerant of heat. His hay fever is therefore eased by cool air, as long as it is not pollen laden.

A dosage regimen for each of these three medicines for hay fever symptoms is one tablet three times daily for 2–3 days as required.

Summary

Hay fever:

- In a chilly, fussy, anxious child with burning discharges – *Ars. alb.* 30C.
- In a chilly, fussy child with bland watery discharges – *Nux vom.* 30C.
- In a yielding, sensitive, heat-intolerant child – *Pulsatilla* 30C.
- Dosage – 1 tablet × 3 per day if required.

CHAPTER 5

Homoeopathic Aids for Common Winter Problems

The problems considered in this chapter are some of the disorders commonly associated with winter months although they can occur at any time of the year. Some of them are infections where a prompt use of an appropriate homoeopathic medicine may assist quick relief and avert a need for stronger medication. In other circumstances, when a disease is more established and other treatment is also required, a homoeopathic medicine can often give additional help. The problems considered will be taken in alphabetical order in the hope that this will assist in home prescribing.

Bronchitis

The medicines from our kit likely to be indicated here are *ACONITE, ANTIMONIUM TARTRATE, BRYONIA, KALI BICH.* and *PHOSPHORUS.* The details about the type of chest discomfort, the cough and sputum produced, as well as the general reactions of the patient, can help us select one of them for use.

Aconite 30C is particularly suitable for the early stages of bronchitis when the patient first shows a rise of temperature and complains of chest tightness with a tickling cough. If these symptoms are also accompanied by an increased level of thirst, a restless rather anxious manner and a tendency for the chest to feel warm, we have many of the features that indicate homoeopathic *Aconite* as an appropriate remedy.

When treatment is started very early in their development a useful dosage is one tablet hourly for 4–5 doses.

For symptoms that have persisted for several days further details concerning their characteristics will be needed to help select a suitable homoeopathic medicine.

For instance, bronchitis with copious white sputum associated with loose, rattling breath sounds from a patient who is generally cross or if a child, peevish, suggests a need for *Antimonium tartrate* 30C. Another feature that may guide us to this medicine is the persistence of so much catarrh that it makes the patient feel nauseated.

In contrast to this profile, bronchitis may include a cough that is loose in the mornings but otherwise dry, is associated with a stitching type of pain, comes in bouts with yellowish sputum and is worse for any movement. These are the localized features that indicate *Bryonia* 30C as a homoeopathic prescription. The more general aspects of the profile indicating the need for *Bryonia* are increased thirst, especially for long drinks, irritability and recurrent sighing.

Another symptom picture with bronchitis is a particular tendency to produce very stringy, tough catarrh, or even plugs of it. When this is a marked feature, especially if the cough associated with it is made worse by eating, we have two strong pointers to the use of *Kali bich*.

With the fourth medicine we are considering here, *Phosphorus* 30C, the emphasis is on a tickle type of cough, hoarseness of the voice and soreness or burning sensation in the larynx or trachea, that is the windpipe. When *Phosphorus* 30C is indicated there is also a tendency to nose bleeds; and generally the patient is sensitive, chilly and thirsty. One of the additional signs suggesting a need for homoeopathic *Phosphorus* is the coughing up of blood, known as haemoptysis. If this happens a medical assessment is needed urgently.

For each of these four medicines in bronchitis, whether they are used as the main prescription or alongside other forms of medicine, a useful dosage regimen is one tablet three times daily for 3–4 days if required.

Summary

Bronchitis:
- Early, with temperature, tight chest, tickle cough, thirst – *Aconite* 30C 1 tablet hourly × 4-5 if required.
- With copious, loose white sputum, rattling cough, peevish – *Ant. tart*. 30C 1 tablet × 3 daily 3-4 days if required.
- With dry, painful cough, thirst and irritability – *Bryonia* 30C 1 tablet × 3 daily 3-4 days if required.
- With stringy catarrh, cough worse for eating – *Kali bich*. 30C 1 tablet × 3 daily 3-4 days if required.
- With hoarseness, burning trachea, tickle cough, thirst – *Phosphorus* 30C 1 tablet × 3 daily 3-4 days if required.

Chilblains

For these commonly occurring irritant, tender, reddish coloured nuisances we will consider three of our twenty medicines, namely *CHAMOMILLA, PULSATILLA* and *RHUS TOX*. Here again, an assessment of the localized symptoms and the more general features of the person who has developed them, can guide us to a particular medicine.

Chamomilla 30C is indicated when chilblains are particularly hot, often causing a patient to put his feet out of bed at night in an effort to relieve them. The temperamental features that suggest a need for *Chamomilla* include a tendency to be hasty, irritable and prone to complain. It is as if the mood shows irritability and heat similar to the chilblains, making an impatient patient.

When *Pulsatilla* 30C is indicated again the chilblains are hot and itchy, made worse by heat so that again the patient may put his feet out of bed to cool them. But the general temperament is different. The patient needing *Pulsatilla* is much more yielding, inclined to be moody but easy going, tearful and helped by sympathy. This is a patient whose impatience is shown with quiet sulks rather than overt protests.

The third medicine, *Rhus tox*. 30C is suggested when the chilblains are particularly irritant and have a burning type of pain associated with marked restlessness so that the patient fidgets or recurrently walks around.

Any one of these medicines may be used for chilblains in the 30C potency with one tablet taken three times daily if required.

Summary

Chilblains:

- That are hot and itchy in an irritable complaining patient – *Chamomilla* 30C 1 tablet × 3 daily if required.
- Again worse for heat but in a docile yielding moody patient – *Pulsatilla* 30C 1 tablet × 3 daily if required.
- Burning and very itchy in a restless, fidgety patient – *Rhus tox*. 30C 1 tablet × 3 daily if required.

Colds

The four medicines from our kit considered here are *ARSENICUM ALBUM, MERC. SOL., NATRUM MUR.* and *NUX VOMICA*. The choice of one of these can be assisted by noting the particular features of the catarrh that comes with the cold and the general reaction of the person who has developed the infection.

Arsenicum album 30C is particularly indicated for corrosive or burning catarrh. A thin or watery texture and a tendency for such catarrh to feel hot and corrosive, is a strong indication for homoeopathic *Arsenicum album*. Sometimes the corrosive sensation is such that the eyes generally feel as if they are burning and often the eyelids look red. Another marked local effect in the profile suggesting this medicine is recurrent sneezing. The more generalized features are chilliness, fastidiousness, anxiety and restlessness.

Merc. sol. 30C is indicated when sneezing and the production of copious thick or watery catarrh are again strong features. But here the catarrh is less corrosive and more purulent while the general temperament is hurried and indifferent rather than fussy as with the previous profile.

A need for *Natrum mur.* 30C is suggested by a watery nasal discharge or thick white catarrh but not a lot of sneezing. The general temperament here is that of a fairly solitary person, a loner, one who can be sensitive to noise or other disturbances but is more likely to be quietly cross than to complain.

The fourth profile, suggesting a need for *Nux vomica* 30C, shows a fastidiousness similar to that in the person who may need *Arsenicum album*. But the person needing *Nux vomica* for their cold symptoms also has a watery catarrh, a lot of sneezing and tends to be obstinate and irritable.

All four medicines, when used for cold symptoms, can be taken in the 30C potency with one tablet three times daily if required.

Summary

Colds:

- With corrosive catarrh, heavy sneezing, in a chilly perfectionist – *Arsen. alb.* 30C 1 tablet × 3 daily if required.
- With purulent catarrh, heavy sneezing with hurried indifference – *Merc. sol.* 30C 1 tablet × 3 daily if required.
- With watery or thick white catarrh in a sensitive loner – *Natrum mur.* 30C 1 tablet × 3 daily if required.
- With watery catarrh, heavy sneezing, in an irritable perfectionist – *Nux vomica* 30C 1 tablet × 3 daily if required.

Coughs

Persistent but recently developed coughs that commonly accompany infections such as colds, bronchitis or influenza will be discussed here. This means that there will be some overlap between the paragraphs that particularly focus on those infections and the suggestions to be made here for coughs from these and other causes. This is deliberate as the comments in the sections of this chapter referring to the overall review of the infections and their general effects on people can be augmented by the additional data we will now consider concerning particular types of the cough. Noting the detailed features of a cough can help confirm the choice of a medicine selected for its relevance to the more generalized effects of a disease.

The medicines we will look at here are *ARSENICUM ALBUM, ANTIMONIUM TARTRATE, BRYONIA, NUX VOMICA* and *PHOSPHORUS*.

Arsenicum album 30C is indicated for a hacking, exhausting cough which tends to be worse in the evening or at night. It may be a wheezy type of cough and is characteristically worsened if the patient is exposed to cold air. It may be dry or loose and is often accompanied by a burning sensation in the chest or throat.

For *Antimonium tartrate* 30C the keynote is rattling from the moisture with the cough. This also leads to hoarseness and the feeling of the patient that he needs to sit up to make breathing easier. The persistent coughing to try to clear the mucus often makes the larynx, that is the voice box, feel tender.

The cough suggesting a need for *Bryonia* 30C as a homoeopathic medicine is dryish, painful, often occurs in bouts and is notably worse if the patient moves around. It often provokes soreness in the throat or larynx and is associated with stitching pain in the chest or head with the coughing. A feature here is the conflict between feeling a need to take slow deep breaths opposed by pain in doing this and a resulting shallow breathing. There is a marked thirst with the cough but drinking and the movement it involves may be followed by even more coughing.

The cough indicating *Nux vomica* 30C also tends to come in bouts but here it is associated with tickling or roughness in the throat. It is a dry sounding cough, is often accompanied by a bursting type of headache and is characteristically worsened by eating or drinking.

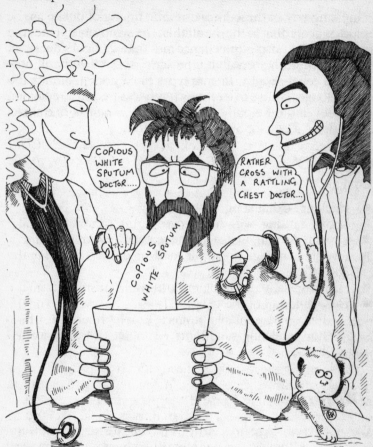

Antimonium tartrate 30C – for coughs

Phosphorus 30C is suggested as a required medicine when the cough is hacking, perhaps even violent and accompanied by chest tightness and burning. Entering a warm room tends to aggravate this cough. The sputum produced is often salty and viscid. The throat sensation is usually tickling, burning or scraping. Although the patient with this type of cough may feel particularly thirsty, drinking often worsens rather than relieves it.

In using any of these medicines the timing of doses can be selected according to the duration of the symptoms. If they are of very recent onset, for instance less than 24 hours duration, one tablet hourly, repeated if required about 4–5 times, may give the relief sought. If symptoms have persisted for a few days a longer course of treatment with less frequent repetition is usually more helpful. A suggested regimen is one tablet three times a day for 3–4 days if required.

Summary

Cough:

- Hacking, exhausting, with burning – *Ars. alb*. 30C.
- Loose, rattling, with hoarseness – *Ant. tart*. 30C.
- Dryish, painful, worse for movement – *Bryonia* 30C.
- Dryish, tickling, worse for food or drink – *Nux vomica* 30C.
- Hacking, salty, scraping or burning – *Phosphorus* 30C.
- Dosage for all of these:
  For very recent symptoms – 1 tablet hourly × 4–5.
  For persisting symptoms – 1 tablet × 3 daily for 3–4 days.

Influenza

We need first here to clarify how we are using the term influenza. Although the symptoms to which it refers are well documented in medical books, in day-to-day use the term is often loosely applied to various medical problems with ill health and a cough. When we discuss it here we will be refering to the combination of general ill health and a rise of temperature, with headache, back and limb aching and usually a harsh dry cough. For this collection of symptoms we will consider using *ACONITE, ARSENICUM ALBUM, BELLADONNA, GELSEMIUM* and *NUX VOMICA*.

The prescribing profile for *Aconite* 30C correlates well with all the features of influenza which we have already summarized. It is particularly indicated for the early stages of a feverish illness when the patient is generally restless or anxious with his or her symptoms, is thirsty but does not feel better for drinking, is flushed but tends to shiver. The headache has a bursting quality, and the aching of the limbs is as if they are bruised. There is often a tickling type of cough.

When *Arsenicum album* 30C is indicated the general profile includes a high level of anxiety and restlessness, especially at night. There is marked thirst, but the symptoms are not relieved by drinking. The general weakness is severe and the pains often burning in character although the patient feels cold. The cough is usually hacking and associated with dryness or burning discomfort of the throat and larynx.

The influenza type symptoms that suggest *Belladonna* 30C as an appropriate remedy again include marked general restlessness and a flushed, hot-looking face. The eyes often take on a staring quality and the pupils appear dilated. The headache tends to be throbbing in quality, the backache a burning discomfort. The thirst may be increased or decreased. The cough is usually short and dry. The keynotes here are anxiety, restlessness and flushing.

Gelsemium 30C is a medicine widely useful for the heavy, wearisome, aching type of influenza. There is less emphasis on restlessness in this prescribing profile, more on tiredness, apathy and irritability. It is the sort of influenza where the patient feels too weary to get up. The headache tends to be dull and heavy, the cough dry, the throat dry with burning discomfort and the limbs aching with a heavy feeling and easily tired by slight exercise.

For *Nux vomica* 30C the prescribing profile includes particular emphasis on coldness and irritability. The more specific symptoms of influenza that suggest *Nux vomica* are a dry or tickling cough that is worsened by eating or drinking, a heavy or pressing type of headache, especially over the eyes, and a bruised aching sensation of the back and limbs. But the more generalized features remain the common strong lead to

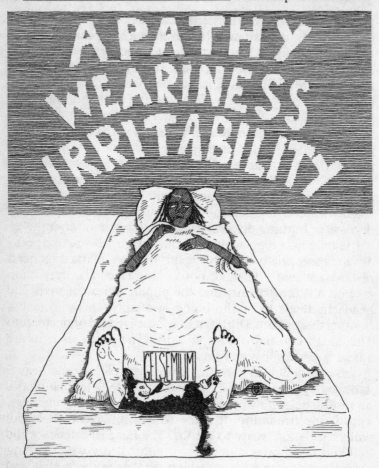

Gelsemuim 30C – for flu

a prescription of *Nux vomica* 30C with their emphasis on fussiness, irritability and obstinacy. This medicine is sometimes briefly depicted as one for harassed businessmen. If this short but telling description applies now to a patient who also has the particular symptoms of influenza, this medicine can be á useful aid.

For all such influenzal type reactions a suggested dosage for these medicines is one tablet of the 30C potency taken hourly for 3-4 doses for very recently developed symptoms, or three times daily for 3-4 days for those of longer duration.

Summary

Influenza:

- With restless apprehension, flushed, shivering - *Aconite* 30C.
- With restless anxiety, burning pains, coldness - *Ars. alb.* 30C.
- With flushing, throbbing headache, restlessness - *Belladonna* 30C.
- With general apathy, weariness and irritability - *Gelsemium* 30C.
- With irritability, obstinacy and coldness - *Nux vom.* 30C.
- Dosage:
  Very recent symptoms - 1 tablet hourly × 3-4 if needed.
  Longer term symptoms - 1 tablet × 3 per day 3-4 days if needed.

Laryngitis

For this common problem three of the medicines from our kit will be discussed: *ACONITE*, *KALI BICH*. and *PHOSPHORUS*.

The type of laryngitis for which *Aconite* 30C is well suited includes a hacking cough with irritant or burning discomfort in the larynx that is worsened by local pressure or coughing. The voice is husky or lost. The general features accompanying this are restlessness, apprehension, chilliness and increased thirst.

A need for *Kali bich.* 30C as a medicine for laryngitis is indicated when the local effects include roughness of the voice and the production of particularly stringy catarrh which is difficult to clear. The pain is more of a rawness. When these local features are present they are often a sufficient guide in themselves to a successful prescription of *Kali bich*. The general features that may also endorse the use of this medicine are tiredness, or weary irritability.

With the type of laryngitis indicating a need for *Phosphorus* 30C the emphasis is again on roughness of the voice but here the local pain is more of a burning quality which is worsened by talking or coughing and at times feels as if it is a grasping of the larynx. Local pressure makes the symptoms worse. There is an increased thirst, particularly for cold drinks, but these do not relieve the symptoms. In general *Phosphorus* is particularly suited to chilly people who easily become sad and are highly sensitive.

Summary

Laryngitis:

- Voice lost, burning discomfort, hacking cough – *Aconite* 30C.
- Rough voice, very stringy mucus, tiredness – *Kali bich* 30C.
- Rough voice, burning pain, worse for talking – *Phosphorus* 30C.
- Dosage – 1 tablet = 3 per day for 2–3 days as required.

Sinusitis

Two medicines that have often helped patients with sinusitis and are included in our kit are *KALI BICH.* and *MERC. SOL.*

Kali bich. 30C is particularly indicated for sinusitis associated with stitching type of pain especially in the region of the cheek bones or a pressure sensation at the bridge of the nose. One of the features of pain suggesting a need for *Kali bich.* is for it to occur in small areas so that patients say, for instance, they feel they could put a fingertip on the point of pain. Stooping or movement tend to worsen the pain. The other prominent feature suggesting a need for *Kali bich*. is the

Kali Bichromicum 30C – for sinusitus

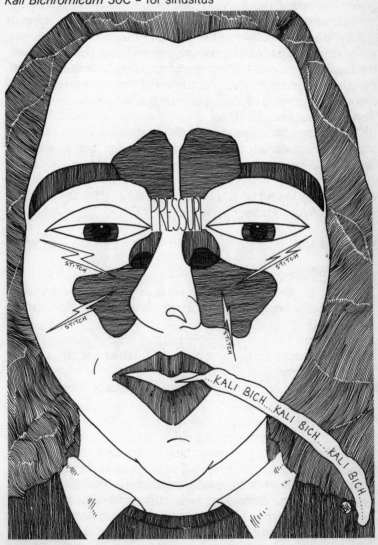

production of thick, stringy, yellow-green catarrh. This often runs down the back of the nose to the throat and is difficult to clear.

A prescription of *Merc. sol.* 30C is more likely to help when the prescribing profile includes a drawing or tearing type of facial pain, particularly in the cheeks, which tends to be worse from exposure to cold air or dampness. The associated catarrh is usually purulent, offensive and copious. Another keynote feature suggesting *Merc. sol.* as an appropriate medicine is profuse salivation and a soft tongue which easily shows indentations from teeth.

The dosage for these medicines for sinusitis again depends on the duration of the symptoms. If they are recent, for instance developing a few hours previously, a useful dosage is 1 tablet hourly for 3–4 doses if required. For symptoms present for a longer time, 1 tablet three times daily for 3–4 days is more likely to help.

Summary

For sinusitis:

- With stringy catarrh, small areas of pain – *Kali bich*. 30C.
- With purulent catarrh, heavy saliva, soft tongue – *Merc. sol*. 30C.
- Dosage:
  For very recent symptoms – 1 tablet hourly × 3–4 if required.
  For longer term symptoms – 1 tablet × 3 per day 3–4 days if required.

Tonsillitis

Suggestions of prescriptions useful for tonsillitis have been discussed in Chapter 4 in relation to disorders commonly shown by children. The data given there apply similarly for tonsillitis occurring in adults and at any time of the year.

CHAPTER 6

Homoeopathic Aids for Common Problems on Holiday

The aim in this chapter is to consider the uses of homoeopathic medicines for the types of problems that often develop in holidays wherever they are taken. These will be considered in two groups, looking first at the difficulties that commonly occur with travelling. This will include anxiety reactions before departure, such as fear of flying, and then problems that occur during the journey such as travel sickness, flight-induced deafness and the difficulties that can arise with over-tired children, or adults. The second section will look at the problems that commonly occur at the holiday destination, considering bowel disorders, digestive upsets and adverse effects from the sun.

For the journey

Travel phobias

Many, or perhaps even most people, experience some anxiety over flying. But for some people the fear prior to or during a flight can be intense and very unpleasant for them. Homoeopathic medicines from our kit that may help here are *ARGENTUM NITRICUM, ARSENICUM ALBUM and* GELSEMIUM. Each of these may be of some help with such anxiety reactions; the particular one to be used can be selected on the overall reactions of the people concerned and how they show their anxieties.

Argentum nitricum 30C is indicated for a person who has diarrhoea with their anxiety, trembles with their fear, has a hurried manner and is noticeably worse in a warm room or environment. Another pointer can be that they crave sweet things but feel worse or get more diarrhoea from eating them.

In contrast to this profile the person who is more likely to find *Arsenicum album* 30C helpful is chilly, fussy and restless. Although they easily feel cold and are improved by warmth, they also complain of burning discomfort. The anxiety that this medicine may help is associated with restless pacing around and a fear of death. In someone phobic of flying this may be their basic fear, and *Arsenicum album* 30C may be a useful aid to help them overcome or at least reduce the reaction.

When *Gelsemium* 30C is indicated the reaction is more subdued. There is irritability and fear of being left alone, but with this there is more emphasis on weakness and lethargy. The physical effects accompanying the anxiety commonly converge on the throat area with a sensation of a lump there and may lead to difficulty with swallowing or speaking.

For each of these medicines a useful dosage is one tablet of the 30C potency taken three times daily prior to the journey or 2 hourly during it.

Summary

Travel anxiety:

- With diarrhoea, worse for warmth and sugar – *Arg. nit.* 30C.
- With restlessness, worse for cold – *Ars. alb.* 30C.
- With weakness, lethargy and throat tension – *Gels.* 30C.
- Dosage for all of these:
  Pre-journey – 1 tablet × 3 per day if required.
  During journey – 1 tablet 2 hourly if required.

Travel sickness

One of three medicines from our kit can be appropriate when children or adults develop sea, car or air sickness. They are *ARNICA, NUX VOMICA* and *STAPHISAGRIA.*

When travel nausea or sickness is associated with tiredness from travelling, *Arnica* 30C can be a useful help. It is particularly indicated for people who are agitated and restless with their nausea and weariness. It is as if they have been over-stimulated by the journey, cannot settle down so keep on fidgeting or wandering around while appearing irritable and grumpy.

When *Nux vomica* 30C is more likely to help with travel sickness, there is again an emphasis on irritability but here the person suffering the problem is more likely to be chilly, fussing about arrangements and cross with themselves or even angry about being nauseated. The particular type of nausea likely to be helped by *Nux vomica* 30C is one where the patient wants to vomit and feels they will be much better for doing so, but finds it difficult. Another time when *Nux vomica* 30C is particularly useful is for travel sickness occurring after overeating a few hours before the journey.

Staphisagria 30C is the third medicine to consider here. It is more useful for nausea occurring before any vomiting develops and for people who have been irritable or even angry over the journey but have kept this mostly to themselves. When someone shows such suppressed anger, and perhaps becomes quietly cross or gloomy if travel plans have not worked out as expected, and this leads onto nausea, *Staphisagria* 30C may well be a useful aid for his humour as well as his stomach.

For all such instances a suggested dosage is one tablet of the 30C potency started as soon as symptoms begin and repeated hourly if required. For individuals who recurrently have travel sickness, if one of these medicines appears likely to suit the symptoms they commonly develop, a single dose taken as the journey starts may help reduce or perhaps prevent the difficulties developing.

Summary

For travel sickness:

- In overtired, fractious person – *Arnica* 30C.
- In cold, fussy, over-fed person – *Nux vom*. 30C.
- With quiet anger and frustration – *Staphisagria* 30C.
- Dosage for all of these – 1 tablet hourly as required.

Flight-induced deafness

These comments refer to the impairment of hearing that often develops during a flight, especially as an aircraft descends, in people with normally healthy ears and hearing. It can be a common nuisance even for people who travel by air when they do not have any obvious catarrhal symptoms. A medicine found useful on several occasions for such problems is *KALI BICH*. 30C. One tablet taken at 30-minute intervals for one or two doses has often been found helpful.

Summary

Flight-induced hearing reduction – *Kali bich*. 30C 1 tablet ½ hourly × 1-2.

Overtired children

Although children are more likely to show the effects of being overtired far quicker than most adults, and this section is therefore focused on their needs, the comments and suggestions made can be applied for people of all ages. Three medicines to consider using here are *ARNICA, BRYONIA* and *NUX VOMICA*. The general demeanour of the child who is overtired can help us select one of these three for use. By this I mean the reaction of the child at the time when they are showing the effects of tiredness. It illustrates the principle discussed in the early chapters introducing homoeopathy, that the prescription of the medicines is frequently made according to the overall presentation of the patient at the time he or she needs it.

Arnica 30C is suited to the child who is like an overwound toy with marked restlessness and achieving little except perhaps the aggravation of other people. It is the sort of restlessness that leads a person to move around frequently, wanting change for the sake of change but with no other clear purpose. The related temperament is agitated, quarrelsome and at times tearful.

Bryonia 30C is more likely to help when the overall profile is one of irritability again, but more discouragement and a greater stubbornness. They are worse for getting cold, are often thirsty and although they are restless and inclined to move around, feel worse for doing so.

Nux vomica 30C also suits the person who is worse for getting cold, but here the demeanour is more fussy and fault finding. The complaints about circumstances while travelling are readily made, especially as the tiredness increases.

A suggested dosage for each of these medicines in this situation is one tablet of the 30C potency ½ hourly if required for up to four doses.

Summary

For overtiredness:

- With non-directed restlessness – *Arnica* 30C.
- With chilliness, irritability and discouragement – *Bryonia* 30C.
- With chilliness, fault finding, fussy behaviour – *Nux vomica* 30C.
- Dosage – 1 tablet ½ hourly up to × 4 if required.

For the holiday

Having started with needs likely to arise with the journey, we now look at some of the common problems encountered while at the place of holiday. We will take them in three groups. First bowel upsets, second digestive problems and third adverse effects of exposure to sun.

Bowel upsets

When the bowel habit, that is the frequency or consistency of stools passed, changes because of the different type of diet eaten during a holiday, appropriate homoeopathic medicines may help towards quick relief. Sometimes these effects clear with the homoeopathic help, but if diarrhoea or vomiting does not improve quickly it is usually advisable to seek professional medical help concerning the possible need for other forms of medicine that may also be required.

I will look first at homoeopathic help for constipation or diarrhoea, and secondly at medicines suitable for the combination of diarrhoea and vomiting.

Constipation or diarrhoea

Such changes commonly occur with the changes of diet when on holiday, especially if we are travelling abroad. Four medicines that we can consider using for either constipation or diarrhoea are *ARSENICUM ALBUM, BRYONIA, NATRUM MUR* and *NUX VOMICA*. Each of these medicines can be appropriate aids for particular types of people with diarrhoea or constipation. The individualizing features both of the person and their bowel difficulties thus need to be noted to select one of these four medicines.

Arsenicum album 30C is indicated when the diarrhoea or constipation is accompanied by burning and slightly colicky abdominal discomfort. The diarrhoea is likely to be profuse and may also lead to local soreness around the anus. The constipation is associated with ineffectual urging as if the bowel is ready to clear, but without result. Generally the person needing *Arsenicum album* 30C is restless, anxious, chilly, particularly concerned that the bowel upset might disrupt their carefully worked out schedule and thirsty for sips of water.

The local symptoms that suggest a need for *Bryonia* 30C are constipation with large bulky stools that feel difficult to pass or loose offensive diarrhoea of undigested food, with either of these types of change provoked particularly by travelling. The more general aspects of the individual profile that are an indication for homoeopathic *Bryonia* are irritability, a tendency to be morose, especially with the bowel complaints and a marked thirst for long drinks.

The features indicating a need for *Natrum mur.* 30C include a strong reaction to salt, either in the atmosphere during a seaside holiday, or in the cooking. When a person develops bowel or other upsets following exposure to salty air or from food that for them is unusually salty, homoeopathic *Natrum mur.* may be of help in assisting a return to order. The bowel upsets that are particularly responsive to this medicine are a watery diarrhoea or the passing of crumbling, dry constipated faeces. The general features that may accompany such local effects, and further suggest a need for this medicine, are a contained irritability, a tendency to brood over problems, easily provoked tiredness and a dislike of heat.

The fourth medicine we are considering here is *Nux vomica* 30C. This is particularly suited to either diarrhoea or constipation provoked by rich or fatty meals in a person known to have difficulty tolerating them. If a watery diarrhoea or dry constipation are obviously linked to these changes of diet or alcohol intake it is worth considering using *Nux vomica* 30C to help reduce the problems. Another physical change that suggests a need for this medicine is the aggravation of haemorrhoids with pain or irritation from the bowel effects. The general features that indicate its use are fussy irritability increased by the bowel problems.

The dosage for any of these prescriptions is determined according to the timing of the bowel symptoms. When they are of recent onset and acute, for instance diarrhoea quickly developing after unsuitable food, one tablet may be required half hourly for 3-4 doses. If the effects have developed gradually over a holiday a helpful dosage is more likely to be one tablet three times daily as required.

Summary

For diarrhoea or constipation:

- With burning discomfort, anal soreness, coldness – *Arsen. album* 30C.
- With bulky stool or offensive diarrhoea, irritability – *Bryonia* 30C.
- Bowel upset from salt, heat intolerance, brooding – *Natrum mur* 30C.
- Fussy irritability and bowel changes from diet or alcohol – *Nux vomica* 30C.
- Dosage:
  Very recent symptoms – 1 tablet ½ hourly × 3–4
  With gradual onset – 1 tablet × 3 per day as required.

Diarrhoea and vomiting

If these occur together they often indicate an infection of the digestive tract. If the symptoms are not too severe and treated early enough a homoeopathic medicine may be followed by quick improvement. If that does not happen and such symptoms persist medical help is advisable and perhaps additional treatment. So we are thinking here of symptoms of recent onset where the person is not dehydrated or obviously ill enough to need more than first aid.

For acute diarrhoea and vomiting of this type two medicines from our kit that may be indicated are *Argentum nitricum* and *Arsenicum album*.

The person likely to be helped by *Argentum nitricum* 30C has flatulence, vomiting and passes very loose or even watery diarrhoea which may be greenish. These problems are often worse for excitement or anticipation of a special activity. They also tend to be worse for warmth. A particular feature suggesting a need for this medicine is a strong desire for sweets but an adverse reaction to them, so that if eaten they aggravate the bowel upset. Another lead to this medicine is the tendency for drinks to cause a quick worsening of the diarrhoea so that they appear to rush through the gastrointestinal tract.

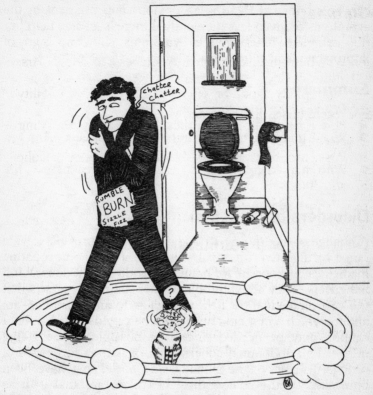

Arsenicum Album 30C – for diarrhoea and vomiting

The profile is different when *Arsenicum album* 30C is more likely to help correct diarrhoea and vomiting. Here there is marked chilliness with the patient looking cold and shivery. Despite this emphasis on coldness the patient is also likely to complain of burning discomfort in the throat, abdomen or rectum. When these local effects are accompanied by marked weakness and restlessness, *Arsenicum album* 30C is strongly indicated.

When such symptoms are acute and recently developed, for instance within the last few hours, a useful dosage is one tablet of the 30C potency hourly for 4–5 doses as required. The dose can be stopped if there is an obvious improvement in the symptoms or given less frequently if there is a some help but not complete relief. If the symptoms show no sign of improving medical help is advisable.

Summary

For recent onset diarrhoea and vomiting:

● Worse for excitement, warmth, drinks or sweets – *Arg. nit.* 30C.
● With marked coldness, restless anxiety, weakness – *Ars. alb.* 30C.

Disorders of digestion

A change of diet during a holiday can easily provoke a wide range of digestive upsets. I will look at the homoeopathic medicines appropriate for flatulence, indigestion, nausea and hangovers. They are all problems that commonly arise when the gastrointestinal tract tries to adjust to an unfamiliar diet and for which a first-aid remedy can be very useful. A note of caution may be needed since it is possible for persisting indigestion, abdominal colicky pain or nausea to be due to serious diseases of the stomach and bowel that have been unmasked by the change of diet. This means that if these symptoms are severe and persistent it is wiser to have a medical check rather than simply continuing with first aid. The need for this is rare and in most instances the sort of problems considered here can be effectively helped by appropriate first-aid measures.

Flatulence

An excess of wind can easily cause unpleasant griping pains or an uncomfortable distension in the abdomen. Two medicines from our kit that may help relieve this are *ARGENTUM NITRICUM* and *ARSENICUM ALBUM*.

The particular features of the abdominal discomfort that

suggest *Argentum nitricum* 30C as the medicine likely to help are griping pains that feel as if a band is pulled tight or a sensation of tremor affecting the stomach or bowel. It may also be compared to the feeling of a ball of pressure within the abdomen and is worsened by minor degrees of external pressure so that even loose clothing becomes uncomfortable. These local complaints are characteristically worse if the person is in a warm room or bed or if they have sweet drinks or food.

Arsenicum album 30C is also suitable for the abdomen that feels generally tight with wind that is difficult to clear. But here the particular effects in the abdomen are a burning discomfort or similarly burning sensation when wind breaks from the stomach with some fluid reflux towards the throat. The burning sensation that we have often noticed as a feature when *Arsenicum album* 30C has been indicated for other problems is again strongly in evidence here. The associated pains from wind are also often like cramp. The general features that suggest a need for this medicine are overall coldness despite the burning discomfort, marked restlessness and anxiety.

With either of these medicines a suggested dosage is one tablet of the 30C potency repeated 2 hourly as required.

Summary

Flatulence:

- With band-like pain or trembling sensation, worse for warmth – *Argentum nit*. 30C.
- With burning discomfort and regurgitation, worse for cold – *Arsenicum alb*. 30C.
- Dosage – 1 tablet 2 hourly as required.

Indigestion

ARGENTUM NITRICUM and *ARSENICUM ALBUM* may again be considered here. The indications are similar to those described in the suggestions on first aid for flatulence with the additional features referring to details of the type of indigestion.

Argentum nitricum 30C is indicated for indigestion provoked by a surge of emotion and accompanied by slight nausea with frequent belching.

The indigestion suggesting a need for *Arsenicum album* 30C is accompanied by marked nausea and burning discomfort that perhaps unexpectedly is worse for cold drinks, more likely helped by hot ones and is characteristically worse around midnight.

Two other medicines to consider here are *NUX VOMICA* and *PULSATILLA*.

Nux vomica 30C is particularly suitable for heartburn with a scraping, raw sensation especially when this follows unsuitable meals eaten far too quickly. The particular provocations of the indigestion suited to this medicine include alcohol, fatty or rich food. When this is the cause, and the problem occurs in a chilly, irritable, fussy and rather pedantic person, *Nux vomica* 30C has good chance of helping the indigestion.

In contrast to this *Pulsatilla* 30C is more suited to a yielding, sensitive, easily impressionable person who feels worse for heat. Other distinguishing features here are the relative lack of thirst, a particular tendency to indigestion after eating fatty food such as pork and a tendency for the patient to feel self-pity.

A suggested dosage with each of these four medicines used for recently developed indigestion is one tablet of the 30C potency repeated half hourly if required.

Summary

Indigestion:

- Worse for heat, sweets and after emotional upsets – *Arg. nit*. 30C.
- With shivering but burning discomfort worse for cold drink – *Ars. alb*. 30C.

- With coldness, worse for fast unsuitable food, fussiness – *Nux vom*. 30C.
- Worse for heat in a sensitive, moody thirstless person – *Pulsatilla* 30C.
- Dosage – if taken soon after onset, 1 tablet ½ hourly × 3–4.

Nausea

The complaint 'I feel sick' is commonly heard during holidays. Children often seem particularly susceptible to the effects of diet change which may be further aggravated by over-excitement. Although perhaps more common in children, this problem can also be shown by adults. The two medicines considered here, *NUX VOMICA* and *PULSATILLA*, are appropriate for all ages.

Nux vomica 30C is particularly suitable for the nausea that comes on quickly after eating, is worse if a person moves around or has recently been travelling, provokes the feeling that vomiting would bring quick relief and with women or girls is coincident with the menstrual period. Generally the person needing *Nux vomica* 30C is likely to be chilly, cross and fussy, with these traits heightening their irritation over changes of plans resulting from the nausea.

Pulsatilla 30C is also an appropriate medicine for nausea developing quickly after eating, especially following rich or fatty food or if it is worse for warm drinks. It is often accompanied by catarrhal conditions and is provoked by excitement. The reaction here is worsened by warmth; the person usually wants cool fresh air for relief. The general features suggesting a need for homoeopathic *Pulsatilla* are a yielding, tearful disposition with an obvious preference for lots of sympathy over the nausea.

For dosage here one tablet of the 30C potency repeated half hourly if required for 3–4 doses.

Summary

Nausea:

- Soon after eating, feels vomiting would help, worse with period and for cold, fussy irritable person – *Nux vom*. 30C.
- After fatty or rich food, warm drinks, excitement, with catarrh in moody person who wants sympathy – *Pulsatilla* 30C.
- Dosage – 1 tablet ½ hourly × 3-4 if required.

Hangovers

A common problem that can occur at any time, but as it may be more likely on holidays it is included here. A remedy often found useful for the irritability, nausea and tense headache

Nux Vomica 30C – for hangover

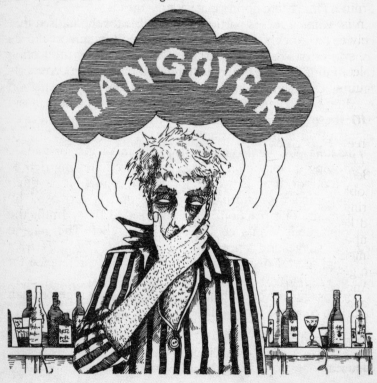

that can follow alcohol intake is *NUX VOMICA* 30C. A useful dosage has been one tablet taken hourly if required. One or two doses are often enough to help relieve such difficulties.

Effects of exposure to sun

Sunburn

Two medicines from our kit that may be considered for skin burning following over-exposure to sun are *BELLADONNA* and *CANTHARIS*. The local effects of the sun on the skin can be a guide to selecting one or other of these medicines.

With any sunburnt skin there is likely to be obvious redness, perhaps slight puffy swelling and generally soreness and burning. *Cantharis* 30C is particularly useful when the skin pain is stinging as well as burning. *Belladonna* 30C is more likely to help when the pain includes throbbing and heat.

A suggested dosage for either of these medicines is one tablet of the 30C potency repeated half-hourly for 3–4 doses if required.

Sun-induced headache

Three medicines from our kit relevant here are *BELLADONNA, BRYONIA* and *PULSATILLA*.

Belladonna 30C is likely to help when there is a pounding or throbbing headache which is worsened by lying flat, stooping, jarring or sudden movement but eased by sitting propped up and keeping the head still or holding it firmly. The overall temperament or mood change indicating a need for homoeopathic *Belladonna* is irritability that increases as the sun gets hotter.

Another medicine that is often helpful for a sun-induced headache is *Bryonia* 30C. This too is useful for a headache which is worse for movement and eased by local pressure. The type of pain for which *Bryonia* is likely to help is compressive or hammering. It is also distinguished by its tendency to be eased by lying flat. The accompanying general reactions include being irritable, thirsty and chilly, although the headache is worse for heat.

A third medicine from our kit that can be useful here is *Pulsatilla* 30C. This is particularly indicated for a dull headache, one that feels as if the head is congested. It is likely to be eased by gentle movement in cool air. The coincident mood changes that suggest a need for *Pulsatilla* include a tendency to be easily upset and tearful, being easily discouraged and wanting sympathy for the headache.

When either of these three medicines are used for sun headaches, a useful dosage is one tablet taken half-hourly 3–4 times if required.

Summary

Sunburnt skin:

- With stinging pain – *Cantharis* 30C.
- With throbbing pain – *Belladonna* 30C.

Headache from too much sun:

- Throbbing with general irritability, crossness – *Belladonna* 30C.
- Compressive, eased by lying flat, thirsty – *Bryonia* 30C.
- Dull with discouragement and tearfulness – *Pulsatilla* 30C.
- Dosage – 1 tablet ½ hourly × 3–4 if required.

Cold sores (herpes simplex)

These unpleasant eruptions often occur on the lips of people prone to them when they are exposed to strong sun or sea air.

A medicine in our kit particularly suitable for such effects of exposure to sea air is *NATRUM MUR.* 30C. For people where the typical herpes simplex eruptions, sometimes known as cold sores, develop when they are on the coast or travelling by sea, this can be a useful aid. A useful regimen is to start taking the medicine as soon as the blister-like eruption starts to develop and continue it three times a day if required for 3–4 days. The use of this medicine has often been associated with the blisters subsiding far quicker than if left untreated.

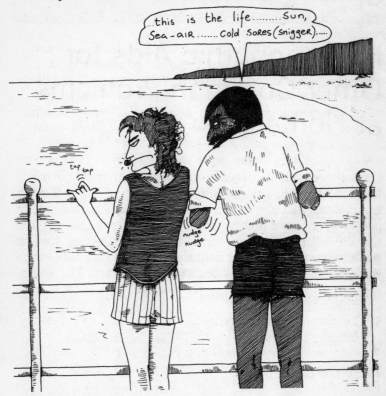

Natrum Muriaticum 30C – for cold sores

Not all such eruptions occur in sea air. Another medicine from our kit to consider when the salt provocation is not present is *Rhus tox*. 30C. This too is likely to be more helpful if started at the first sign of the blisters forming and taken three times daily for 3-4 days as required.

Summary

Herpes, cold sores, on the lips:

- From sea air - *Nat. mur*. 30C.
- Not provoked by salt - *Rhus tox*. 30C.

CHAPTER 7

Homoeopathic Aids for Other Common Problems at Home

Having previously considered a variety of first aid needs likely to occur in particular situations we come now to the sort of problems that can arise in many places and particularly at home. In hopes of making these notes easier to use, the first section will refer to symptoms commonly affecting specific parts of the body starting with the head and headaches then working down to the legs with calf muscle cramps. The second section will refer to more generalized problems such as boils and insomnia.

Headache

Several of the medicines in our kit may be used to ease headaches. One way of selecting just one medicine for use is to start off by considering the type of head pain occurring.

Burning or throbbing discomfort

Two of our medicines to choose between here are *ARSENICUM ALBUM* and *BELLADONNA*.

A particular local feature in addition to the burning or throbbing type of pain that suggests a need for *Arsenicum album* 30C is that the discomfort is briefly eased by placing something cold like a cool damp flannel on the head. The more general aspects of the profile that further suggest this as a useful medicine are restless fussy behaviour, coldness and weakness, but despite these features relief of the pain when walking in cool air.

Belladonna 30C, another medicine we can consider for a burning or throbbing headache, has the local feature that the pain is eased by pressing on the head and sitting up, but is worse for lying flat. More generalized features are a tendency to be much worse for any movement, sudden noise or strong light.

Bursting or splitting headache

Again there are two medicines from our kit to consider, *BRYONIA* and *CHAMOMILLA*.

Bryonia 30C is often a useful aid for headaches of this type which are also markedly worse for any movement so that the patient demands to lie down. Stooping is particularly aggravating here, making this type of headache a lot worse. Noise also makes it worse but firm pressure on the head sometimes helps. In general this patient is cross, fed up and thirsty.

Chamomilla 30C is indicated when a bursting or splitting headache is accompanied by irritability to the extent of rudeness to anyone trying to help. The pain is worsened by warmth or coldness. It is the situation where it is hard to find anything that will please the sufferer who therefore complains frequently about intolerable difficulties.

Dull, heavy headache

There are three medicines that can be appropriate here: *GELSEMIUM, KALI BICH.* and *NUX VOMICA*.

Gelsemium 30C is appropriate for this type of headache when it occurs with pain in the neck and giddiness. The general mood changes that suggest a need for this medicine are irritability or general weariness. Often the patient needing this medicine looks very weary with a tendency to drooping eyelids.

The indications for *Kali bich*. 30C are a dull, heavy headache with pain in localized areas, such as over one eye, or a pain that someone says he can locate with one finger. It is also particularly useful for relief of pain associated with catarrhal congestion or sinusitis, especially if the discomfort is eased by local pressure or lying down.

The third medicine to consider for the dull heavy type of headache is *Nux vomica* 30C. We have previously noted its usefulness for hangovers, so if that is the cause of the problem, this medicine may well help. Other features suggesting its use are giddiness or nausea with the head discomfort, easing of the pain with rest, but aggravation from excitement, cold or noise. In general, homoeopathic *Nux vomica* is particularly suited to chilly, irritable fussy individuals who complain crossly about their symptoms.

For each of these types of headache and the medicines appropriate for them a useful dosage is one tablet of the 30C potency given as soon as possible after the onset of the symptoms and repeated hourly if required up to three or four times.

Summary

Burning or throbbing headache:

- With fussy restlessness, cold flannel or walking eases – *Ars. alb.* 30C.
- With irritability, lying flat or local pressures eases – *Belladonna* 30C.

Bursting or splitting headache:

- Worse for movement or cold, eased by pressure, lying down – *Bryonia* 30C.
- With rudeness, complaining, intolerance of helpers – *Chamomilla* 30C.

Dull, heavy headache:

- With pain also into neck, giddiness, weary irritability – *Gels*. 30C.
- With catarrh, pain in small areas or over one eye – *Kali bich*. 30C.
- From excitement, irritable, worse for cold and noise – *Nux vom*. 30C.
- Dosage – 1 tablet hourly as required × 3–4.

Eye problems

Eyes are particularly sensitive and complex organs requiring special care to make sure that first aid is correctly used. In many situations such help is highly beneficial. But if symptoms are severe or do not respond quickly to the measures applied it is usually wise to seek medical advice.

Aching eyes

A common complaint which may follow times of intense study or other activity requiring a degree of concentration on close work unusual for the person. In this situation a first-aid remedy may give useful help.

ACONITE 30C is often useful when an aching discomfort of the eyes is accompanied by increase in the flow of tears or watering of the eyes. Other features that suggest *Aconite* as an appropriate homoeopathic medicine here are an increase of the discomfort in strong or bright light and in cold air.

In contrast to this, another medicine that may be helpful, *PULSATILLA* 30C, is sugggested by an aggravation of the aching discomfort with warmth or windy conditions. Again the eyes are prone to water easily, they are also inclined to a smarting discomfort as well as the aching pain.

Conjunctivitis

The type of conjunctivitis considered here is a recently

developed soreness, smarting or gritty sensation in the eyes, with some redness of the eye and sticky discharge. First aid can often be helpful for such symptoms. If the pain is severe or the symptoms have lasted more than a day or two, it is wiser to seek medical help. For first-aid purposes we will consider *ACONITE, ARGENTUM NITRICUM* and *ARSENICUM ALBUM*.

Aconite 30C has already been mentioned in relation to aching eyes. If the features noted there apply again, with the additional signs of early conjunctivitis, *Aconite* 30C may be helpful.

Argentum nitricum 30C is more likely to help when the conjunctival changes are associated with a gritty sensation, sometimes likened to having sand in the eyes, and the symptoms are worse in a warm atmosphere.

When *Arsenicum album* 30C is indicated, the emphasis shifts to burning discomfort in the eyes with burning tears. The eyelids may be swollen and painful with a burning discomfort similar to that affecting the eyes. The symptoms are usually worse in bright light.

Styes

A common problem for which two of our medicines may be helpful. They are *PULSATILLA* and *STAPHISAGRIA*.

Pulsatilla 30C is suited to styes producing a soft whitish/yellowish discharge with marked watering of the eyes and itching as well as stickiness of the lid margins. The person who responds well to homoeopathic *Pulsatilla* is usually moody, easily tearful about the symptoms and wants sympathy and affection. He or she usually likes the open air but soon finds that windy conditions markedly increase the watering of the eyes.

The profile of the person likely to helped by *Staphisagria* 30C has many contrasting features. The localized effects are smarting or aching pain with lid edges that are swollen and producing a more purulent discharge than is likely when *Pulsatilla* is needed. In general a person who needs

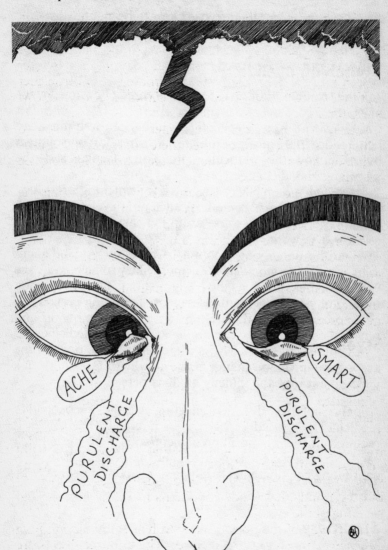

Staphisagria 30C – for styes

Staphisagria 30C for their stye is likely to be gloomy, irritable or angry.

Twitching eyelids

Another common nuisance for which three of our medicines may be considered, namely *ARSENICUM ALBUM*, *CHAMOMILLA* or *PULSATILLA*. Either of these three can help reduce this irritating problem. We can select one of them by observing the particular provoking factors and the associated mood changes.

Arsenicum album 30C is suggested for twitching associated with anxiety or fear. Sometimes twitching eyelids can be a result of generalized tension or apprehension, as if a startle reflex is over-working.

When the underlying emotion is more likely to be anger than anxiety *Chamomilla* 30C is more likely to help. We have noted in other situations the likely role of *Chamomilla* when there is obvious anger and discontent. Twitching eyelids can be another sign of the link between such emotions and physical changes and *Chamomilla* an effective medicine.

In contrast *Pulsatilla* 30C is more likely to help when the accompanying mood change is one of peevish tearfulness in a yielding but probably quietly anxious person.

For each of these disorders affecting eyes the homoeopathic medicines suggested can be given hourly for 3-4 doses if required. If there is no improvement with these measures a careful re-assessment is needed; and particularly if there is continuing conjunctivitis, additional advice and help may be needed.

Summary

Aching eyes:

- Worse for cold and light - *Aconite* 30C.
- Worse for warmth and wind - *Puls.* 30C

Conjunctivitis:

- Soreness and watering, worse in cold – *Aconite* 30C.
- Gritty pain, worse for warmth – *Arg. nit.* 30C.
- Burning pain, stinging tears – *Ars. alb.* 30C.

Styes:

- Sticky eyelids, creamy coloured discharge – *Pulsatilla* 30C.
- Smarting, swollen lid margins, pus discharge – *Staphisagria 30C.*

Twitching lids:

- With anxiety or fear – *Ars. alb.* 30C.
- With anger – *Chamomilla* 30C.
- With peevish tears – *Pulsatilla* 30C.

Dosage: 1 tablet repeated hourly × 3–4 if required.

Mouth disorders

Cracked lips

Cracking of lips, either at the corners of the mouth or around the mid-line, can be a painful nuisance at any time of the year but is particularly common in winter months. Three medicines from our kit to consider for this problem are *BRYONIA, NATRUM MUR.* and *MERC. SOL.*

Bryonia 30C is likely to be a suitable medicine when the cracking is accompanied by a bitter taste in the mouth and a general dryness and burning sensation of the lips. These sensations may contribute to a marked thirst for long drinks which is also a pointer to the use of potentized *Bryonia*.

When *Natrum mur.* 30C is more likely to help the cracks are usually about midway along the lips. Here again the mouth and lips are likely to be generally dry but the distinguishing taste is commonly salty. The emphasis on salt also shows in the factors likely to provoke the cracking, *Natrum mur.* being particularly helpful when the changes in the lips follow exposure to sea air or extra salty food.

Merc. sol. 30C, in contrast to the previous two medicines, is suited to the treatment of painful cracking of the lips when the mouth is generally moist, with copious saliva. This may be sufficiently marked for there to be obvious dribbling. Cracks at the corners of the mouth and a soft, flabby looking tongue so that it looks as if the teeth push into its edge, are further guides to the use of *Merc. sol.*

A suggested dosage for the aid of these problems with either of these three medicines is one tablet of the 30C potency two hourly 3–4 times for recent and acute symptoms, or three times daily for 3 days if they have persisted for a few days.

Dental abscess

A medicine in our kit often found helpful for this problem is *Merc. sol.* 30C. It can be used as a first-aid measure while seeking dental treatment or as an adjunct to treatment recommended by a dentist.

Usually such an abscess is associated with some degree of local swelling, pain that may be burning or throbbing in quality and at times seems associated with pain in the ear. One of the features of pain from a dental abscess is that it gets worse after hot drinks, particularly as regards its throbbing nature. Such symptoms have often been eased by taking *Merc. sol.* 30C one tablet 2 hourly for 3–4 doses.

Mouth ulcers

If mouth ulcers are a recurrent problem it is usually wise to seek medical or dental advice about their cause. Even when this is needed we may still find a first-aid medicine helpful while waiting for an appointment. Three medicines to consider here are *ARSENICUM ALBUM, KALI BICH.* and *MERC. SOL.*

Arsenicum album 30C is indicated particularly when ulcers occur on the tongue, often they are on its edges, and they provoke burning pain. There may be a bitter taste in the mouth which is generally dry so that there is moderate thirst.

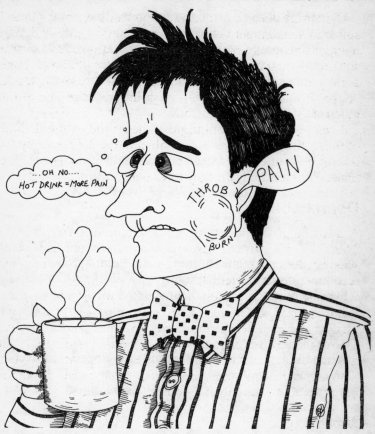

Mercurius Solubilis 30C – for dental abscess

Arsenicum album is further suggested when the pain from ulcers is eased by warm drinks.

Mouth ulcers that suggest *Kali bich*. 30C for their treatment look as if they have yellow slough in their bases and feel firm or thickened to touch. They occur anywhere in the mouth and are likely to be associated with stinging pain. Often there is marked production of stringy saliva that may taste salty.

Merc. sol. 30C is indicated for ulcers that look spongy, yellowish and occur particularly on the palate or tongue in a mouth that looks soft, moist and has gums that bleed easily. Halitosis also suggests a need for *Merc. sol.*

A suggested dosage is one tablet of the 30C potency 2 hourly for acute and newly developed ulcers, one three times daily for 2–3 days if they have occurred a few days before treatment.

Summary

Cracked lips:

- With burning, bitter taste and thirst – *Bryonia* 30C.
- Mid-line, worse from salt air or food – *Nat. mur.* 30C.
- At corners, with moist mouth – *Merc. sol.* 30C

Dental abscess: *Merc. sol.* 30C

Mouth ulcers:

- Especially on tongue, burning pain – *Ars. alb.* 30C.
- Yellow slough in base, stinging – *Kali bich.* 30C.
- Especially tongue and palate, spongy, moist – *Merc. sol.* 30C.

Dosage:

- When these problems have recently developed – 1 tablet 2 hourly × 3–4.
- If present for more than 24 hours pre-treatment – 1 tablet × 3 per day 3–4 days as required.

Voice problems, hoarseness or loss

Four of the medicines from our kit that are indicated for this problem are *ACONITE, ARNICA, KALI BICH.* and *PHOSPHORUS.* The likely causes of the voice changes and the associated general reactions of the patient can help us choose one of them for use. If hoarseness persists, and particularly if it lasts more than 4–5 weeks, it is important to seek specialist medical advice.

Voice changes with laryngitis

When the hoarseness or loss of voice occurs with signs of infection such as slight rise in temperature, general malaise, coughing and throat irritation, a useful aid to treatment is often *Aconite* 30C. The use of this medicine is further supported by restlessness with the complaints, increased level of thirst and brief easing of the throat and voice changes after drinks.

Hoarseness after over-use of the voice

People often become husky or may even lose their voice after using it for longer or more forcefully than is their norm. Examples are voice problems after shouting loud and long at sporting events or having to raise the voice for lectures. In such circumstances a first-aid remedy is *Arnica* 30C.

Hoarseness with catarrh

A persistence of catarrh in the throat or nose after infections such as colds is often associated with voice loss or hoarseness. This suggests a need for *Kali bich.* 30C, particularly if the catarrh is thick, stringy and yellowish.

Another medicine to consider for voice changes in such circumstances is *Phosphorus* 30C. This is more likely to help when the catarrh is associated with burning discomfort in the throat, increased thirst, intermittent bouts of coughing and worsening of all these effects with talking.

A suggested dosage regimen in each of these circumstances is one tablet of the 30C potency of the selected medicine, taken 2 hourly for 3–4 doses if required.

Summary

Hoarseness:

- From over-use of the voice – *Arnica* 30C.
- With laryngitis – *Aconite* 30C.
- From catarrh: thick, stringy – *Kali bich.* 30C.
- With burning throat, thirst – *Phosphorus* 30C.

Abdominal disorders

I have already considered some of the commonly occurring abdominal problems where first aid is appropriate. Chapter 4 referred to medicines likely to help with colic, and Chapter 6 to medicines for diarrhoea, constipation, diarrhoea and vomiting, flatulence, indigestion and nausea. I will now add to this list of abdominally focused disorders by considering ways of helping period pains, known technically as dysmenorrhoea, and cystitis.

Cystitis

Cystitis implies inflammation of the bladder and is usually associated with a need to pass urine more frequently than usual with burning or cutting pain during its passage. Sometimes there is also obvious blood in the urine. If this occurs or if these symptoms are severe or persistent medical advice is also needed. For less severe episodes, or while additional treatment is being sought, a homoeopathic medicine may give useful first aid. The three medicines we will consider here may all be indicated for the local effects in the bladder area and discomfort when passing urine; the selection of one of them can be made by noting the general reaction of the patient.

Three medicines from our kit to consider using here are *CANTHARIS, MERC. SOL.* and *PULSATILLA*.

Cantharis 30C, a medicine widely used in homoeopathy for cystitis, is particularly likely to help when the pain on passing urine is burning in character and the person's reaction to it includes anxious restlessness, crossness and even anger. It is as if the temper burns like the urine passed.

Merc. sol. 30C is indicated when the pain accompanies the passage of urine and then is followed by soreness and continued urging from the bladder. It is as if there is a prolonged urge to keep on passing more urine even though the bladder seems to have been emptied. Perhaps it is not surprising that the mood accompanying such effects is sometimes a weary despondency, as if the patient is thoroughly fed up with it and then shows indifference to those who try to help him or her. A combination of such indifference, despondency and urging suggests the need for *Merc. sol.* 30C.

In contrast to this profile we may see a patient who has the usual symptoms of cystitis but clearly welcomes sympathy offered on account of them. Such patients usually show their feelings readily, perhaps expressing tears as readily as they pass urine with this problem. If such reactions are also accompanied by an intolerance of stuffy heat and a reluctance to drink the extra fluids usually advised when someone has cystitis, *Pulsatilla* 30C is even more strongly indicated as a first-aid remedy.

For dosage with each of these medicines used for acute cystitis, a useful regimen has often been one tablet of the 30C potency taken 2 hourly up to 5–6 times if required.

Period pains (dysmenorrhoea)

Homoeopathic medicines have often been found helpful for this problem. Ideally they are selected after a detailed review of the types of discomfort provoked and the individual features of the physical status and temperament of the person concerned. However, for first-aid purposes when a detailed review is difficult or a trained homoeopathic prescriber is not readily available, use can be made of the salient features shown by the patient to select one of the first-aid medicines from our kit of 20 remedies. We can consider using *BELLADONNA, CHAMOMILLA* and *PULSATILLA*, all in the 30C potency, with the particular type of pain and the main features in the personal reaction to it guiding us to one of these medicines.

Belladonna 30C is particularly indicated when cramp-like pains in the area of the uterus (that is, the womb) come and go suddenly. They may also be associated with a feeling as if the abdominal contents are pressing or dropping down. The general reaction that suggests a need for *Belladonna* 30C is irritable restlessness.

When *Chamomilla* 30C is more likely to help the localized pains are colicky, like a minor version of labour pains, with a tendency for the pain to spread into the thighs or back and to be eased by warmth, for instance from a hot water bottle. The mood changes that suggest a need for this medicine are bad temper or anger. The combination of the local pain and the mood changes may well lead to complaints that the woman's lot is unbearable.

Pulsatilla 30C is more likely to help a rather different type of patient and local discomfort. Here, the general profile is one of tearfulness and sympathy seeking, with local pain in the lower abdomen that may be a pressing ache or crampy colic.

A helpful dosage with any of these medicines is likely to be one tablet of the 30C potency 2–4 hourly up to four times a day as required.

Summary

Cystitis:

- With temper and irritability – *Cantharis* 30C.
- With indifference and recurrent bladder urge – *Merc. sol.* 30C.
- With tears and hopes for sympathy – *Pulsatilla* 30C.
- Dosage – 1 tablet 2 hourly × 5–6 if required.

Period pains:

- Sudden cramps, with irritability – *Belladonna* 30C.
- Like labour, with anger – *Chamomilla* 30C.
- Aching or colicky, tearful, wants sympathy – *Pulsatilla* 30C.
- Dosage – 1 tablet 2–4 hourly or × 4 per day as required.

Limb and back problems

Various types of injury have been considered in Chapter 3. I will add to the limb and back problems considered there by looking at first-aid assistance for calf cramps, thinking particularly of the sort that are often a nuisance at night. For back problems I will look at some aids for pain associated with strain of the type that often follows excessive sport or gardening.

Calf cramps

Sudden cramping pains in the calf muscles as a person settles into bed are a common and very uncomfortable problem that occurs more frequently with increasing age. Rubbing the affected calf muscles often helps release the spasms. Additional help may also be found from taking *Rhus. Tox*. 30C. This medicine may not only help relieve the initial spasm or cramp, but can also reduce the nagging ache that sometimes follows it. A suggested dosage is *Rhus. tox*. 30C one tablet sucked slowly as required.

Backache from over-exertion

Three medicines to consider using here are *ARNICA, BRYONIA* and *RHUS. TOX*. The type of pain and the measures that intensify or relieve it can help us decide on one of them.

Arnica 30C is particularly indicated when backache accompanies bruising or when it feels as if this is the problem even though bruises cannot be seen. It is the reaction that is often experienced after prolonged or unfamiliar exertion leaving the back feeling sore and tender even though no changes can be seen on looking at it. There is accompanying restlessness but continued movement does not relieve the ache or may even make it worse. The pain has been likened to the effect of a hard bed.

The backache that suggests a need for *Bryonia* 30C is definitely worse for movement. This medicine suits the type of back pain accompanied by stiffness that niggles generally but increases with any movement of the area affected so that the patient is likely to lie on the part to keep it fixed and reduce the discomfort.

In contrast to this, the back pain suggesting the use of *Rhus. Tox.* 30C is eased by movement. Here again there may be stiffness with the aching pain but its characteristics include its gradual relief by moving around. The person with this type of pain therefore either paces around, fidgets or recurrently changes position, finding that this gradually reduces the pain.

For use of either of these three medicines a suggested dosage is one tablet of the 30C potency taken hourly if required up to four times for recent-onset problems or one three times daily for 2–3 days if they started more than 24 hours ago.

Summary

Calf cramps – *Rhus. tox.* 30C 1 tablet as required.

Backache from over-exertion:

- As if bruised – *Arnica* 30C.
- Aching and stiffness worse for moving – *Bryonia* 30C.
- Aching and stiffness eased by moving – *Rhus. tox.* 30C.

Dosage:

- Treated early – 1 tablet hourly × 4 if required.
- Treated later – 1 tablet × 3 per day for 2–3 days.

Having considered first aid medicines for some of the problems that can be assessed by looking at parts of the body from head to feet, we come now to more generalized disorders. Here we will look at problems that can arise on almost any particular area of the body, such as boils, or that obviously have generalized effects, such as exam nerves, grief or emotional shock reactions and sleeplessness.

Boils

If boils occur recurrently it is advisable to seek medical advice as eruptions of this type might be an indication of a general disease heightening the chances and severity of local skin infections. Medical help is also usually advised if boils are large or in acutely painful areas such as the ears. But such problems are rare compared with boils which people may treat themselves and where appropriate first-aid medicines can give useful additional help.

Two medicines from our kit to consider using are *BELLADONNA* and *MERC. SOL.* with the stage of the boil needing treatment indicating which to select.

Belladonna 30C is useful for the early stages of development of this localized infection. It is often said that homoeopathic *Belladonna* is appropriate for helping diseases where there is heat, redness, swelling and tenderness. When a boil is in its early stages before the pus comes to a head this description fits it well and implies that *Belladonna* 30C can be an appropriate medical aid.

For the later stages in its development when the pus has obviously started collecting to form a head, more help is likely to be given by *Merc. sol.* 30C. The boil is still likely to be red, tender and generally painful but the addition of the pus forming distinguishes it as a later stage in its development and suggests *Merc. sol.* 30C as a more appropriate medicine.

For dosage of either of these medicines I suggest one 30C potency tablet repeated 2 hourly up six times.

Summary

Boils:

- Early stage – *Belladonna* 30C.
- When head formed – *Merc. sol.* 30C.
- Dosage for either stage 1 tablet 2 hourly × 6 if required.

Exam nerves or anticipatory anxiety

Exams are one cause of anticipatory anxiety. There are of course many others, including driving tests, demanding social functions or interviews and various other events that provoke alarm in the people about to experience them. On many occasions such anxiety reactions have been eased by homoeopathic medicines which also have the additional advantage of not inducing drowsiness.

Three medicines from our kit likely to be helpful here are *ARGENTUM NITRICUM*, *ARSENICUM ALBUM* and *GELSEMIUM*. Anxiety can show itself in various ways and we need to note the details of the reactions provoked to select one of these for use.

Argentum Nitricum 30C – for exam nerves

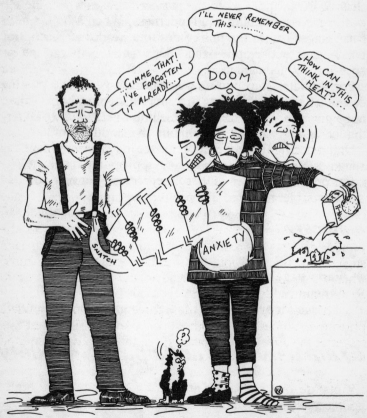

Argentum nitricum 30C is indicated when the person concerned becomes hurried in manner and impulsive in reaction to their apprehension. It is as if they are driven on increasingly faster by the anxiety whirling within and as a result show a lack of concentration which in turn makes them appear forgetful. They are likely to complain of feeling worse for getting warm. Another physical effect of their hurried state can be diarrhoea.

In contrast in some ways, but similar in others, is the profile suggesting a need for *Arsenicum album* 30C. Here again there is restless hurry, but in marked contrast the person is chilly and very fussy. This medicine is more likely to help a person with a perfectionist personality whose anxiety is heightened by a fear of being late or failing to follow a required procedure. Such fear or anxiety may be so intense at times that it leads to apparent indifference to pleasure so that the person cannot even be cheered up by talk of pleasant aspects of a coming event. The thought of a party after the exam or a super honeymoon after a wedding does little to relieve the anxiety that suggests a need for *Arsenicum album* 30C.

Different again is the reaction indicating *Gelsemium* 30C as a medicine more likely to help with anticipatory anxiety. The keynote here is irritability. Often people become irritable when they are anxious. When this is combined with an easy tendency to cry, reactions made worse if the person is alone or moves about, and a dazed or bemused type of response, the profile suggests a need for *Gelsemium* 30C. A further sign suggesting the need for this medicine can be 'exam funk' when the negative reactions lead to the person wanting to back out of the test situation.

For the dosage of either of these three medicines for anxiety prior to examinations, or other special events, I suggest one tablet of the 30C potency taken three times daily as required for up to 3 days.

Summary

Exam nerves:

- With apprehension worse for heat – *Arg. nit.* 30C.
- With fear, restless, worse for cold – *Ars. alb.* 30C.
- With irritability, worse for moving, funk – *Gelsemium* 30C.
- Dosage – 1 tablet × 3 per day for 3 days if required.

Sudden grief and emotional shocks

I am thinking here of the personal reactions to experiences such as sudden frights, for instance after accidents, or the effects from bereavements or other occasions when bad news is received and someone has to cope with a sudden upsurge of emotions. We will be familiar with the range of reactions that such challenges can evoke. The shocked individuals may be quiet, tearful or perhaps angry, but in their differing ways they are responding to a major stress and expressing or restraining the emotional energy provoked. Often a homoeopathic medicine has been a useful aid in such situations.

Relevant medicines from our kit that can be considered for use here are *ACONITE, NATRUM MUR., PULSATILLA* and *STAPHISAGRIA.*

Aconite in the potentized form is mainly helpful for the anxiety and shock that can easily be provoked by sudden frights such as from experiencing personally or seeing a road accident. When after such an experience someone is tearful, anxious, restless and agitated, a prompt use of *Aconite* 30C can often help reduce this surge of reactions and help them settle to a more collected state.

The other three medicines listed above are more likely to help when bad news or other shocks provoke strong surges of emotion such as grief. An example would be a reaction to bereavement or news of another major loss. The details of the reactions evoked can help us select one of these three medicines for use.

Natrum mur. 30C has often been helpful for people reacting to bereavement, particularly when this provokes tears of grief which are then held back until the person can cry alone. This medicine is specially suited to the person who feels worse when others offer consolation so that in public they contain their feelings behind a stiff upper lip. It is a picture of in-held grief, sadness and tiredness.

In contrast to this are people who show their grief readily and even seek support and comfort from those around. For someone reacting in this way, expressing tears readily and welcoming consolation, a helpful homoeopathic medicine is much more likely to be *Pulsatilla*. A further indication for this medicine is a yielding disposition so that the person concerned readily goes along with suggestions about what to do in the situation.

The third of our medicines has yet another very different profile to suggest its use. The indications for *Staphisagria* 30C include an emphasis on an angry reaction. Sometimes bad news or personal shocks can induce anger in the person concerned, shown for instance when they angrily think of blaming themselves or others for the events and express this in their speech and manner. For such surges of anger, which also at times come with tears of grief, *Staphisagria* 30C is likely to be helpful.

A useful dosage for any of these four medicines for such emotional reactions is one tablet of the 30C potency taken hourly if required soon after the shock or news.

Summary

After physical trauma or shock – *Aconite* 30C.

After bad news:

- In-held grief, worse for consolation – *Nat. mur.* 30C.
- Expressed grief, wants consolation – *Pulsatilla* 30C.
- Angry grief and tears – *Staphisagria* 30C.

Dosage – 1 tablet hourly if required for acute reaction up to × 6.

Insomnia (sleeplessness)

BELLADONNA, BRYONIA and *NUX VOMICA* are three medicines from our kit that can be used for first aid here. The details about the likely causes and the type of the sleep difficulty can guide us to choose one of them for use.

The *Belladonna* preparation used in homoeopathic medicine is particularly likely to help sleeplessness associated with anxiety. When anxious thoughts keep churning over making sleep difficult, or when it does come contribute to frightening dreams, *Belladonna* 30C is an appropriate homoeopathic aid. Other features associated with the profile suggesting its use are startled jumpy movements shortly before or during sleep and feeling drowsy but still having difficulty getting to sleep.

The profile for which *Bryonia* 30C is more helpful again includes the tendency to feel sleepy but with difficulty moving from this into sleep. Pressurized thoughts are also another feature here, but this time they are particularly associated with business or family concerns. Dreams similarly tend to be pre-occupied with work. The sleeplessness here is particularly difficult before midnight and worse for heat. Another guide to the need for homoeopathic *Bryonia* is disturbance of sleep by recurrent thirst.

_ *Nux vomica* 30C is more likely to help the sleeplessness that has been contributed to by various excesses. That is, after excessive work when the mind is overtired, or after too much coffee, food or alcohol when the body has had its capacity stretched. This overstretched tendency is also reflected in the poor tolerance of noise so that slight disturbance makes this sort of sleeplessness worse. The sleep or insomnia pattern here is a tendency to get to sleep at first, become wide awake in the very early morning, then feel drowsy and perhaps sleep later so that it becomes difficult to wake and get going for the next day.

A suggested dosage for these medicines for recently developed sleep difficulties is one tablet, repeated if needed an hour later each night for up to three nights a week.

Summary

Sleeplessness:

- With anxiety, tosses around, frightening dreams – *Belladonna* 30C.
- Thinks and dreams of work, worse for heat and thirst – *Bryonia* 30C.
- From over-stimulation, alert in night, drowsy later – *Nux vom*. 30C.
- Dosage – 1 tablet hourly × 2 per night, for 3 nights in week.

CHAPTER 8

Reflections

The use of homoeopathic medicines in first aid has introduced many people to this form of prescribing and has often led them to ask more about it. Three questions are frequently posed:

1. What other medical problems can it be used to treat?
2. How can it be obtained?
3. How does it work?

In this final chapter I will briefly consider these three questions.

First then, for what other diseases can homoeopathic medicines be helpful? The previous chapters have referred to many acute, that is short-lasting diseases, where the use of homoeopathic medicines has often appeared to reduce the severity and duration of symptoms. There are also many chronic, that is long-lasting diseases, where homoeopathic medicines have been found helpful. For several of these diseases homoeopathic medicines may be the only prescription required. But for others it can be used alongisde non-homoeopathic medication, giving additional benefits. For example, problems as diverse as chronic catarrh, migraine, haemorrhoids and hay fever have often been relieved with homoeopathic medicines as the main prescription used. While with other disorders such as asthma, colitis and tumours, the addition of homoeopathic prescriptions has often been associated with an improvement in the person's general level of health and well-being as well as a further reduction of the more localized effects of the diseases so that the need for stronger medication is reduced.

It is often observed that there are two main groups of people seeking homoeopathic treatment. There are those who prefer this system of prescribing and use it as far as possible for all their needs. Another group has their emphasis the other way round. They try other forms of medicine first and only ask for homoeopathy if more conventional lines of treatment fail to give them the help they are seeking. The second group probably constitutes the majority of people referred to homoeopathic outpatient clinics in the National Health Service. Some people from the first group also come to these clinics but the majority are those who have tried other measures, are still having problems so are looking for additional forms of therapy. Even if homoeopathy cannot cure problems such as osteo-arthritis, colitis and tumours, an appropriate use of its medicines may well give additional help to people experiencing them.

In referring to homoeopathic facilities in National Health Service hospitals we are already moving onto the second question often asked: where can advice be found on homoeopathic prescribing? There are five NHS hospital departments offering homoeopathic medicine within the UK. These are in London, Glasgow, Bristol, Liverpool and Tunbridge Wells. The hospitals concerned are The Royal London Homoeopathic Hospital; The Glasgow Homoeopathic Hospital; The Bristol Homoeopathic Hospital; Mossley Hill Hospital, Liverpool; and The Tunbridge Wells Homoeopathic Hospital. Apart from the homoeopathic department in Tunbridge Wells they all offer out-patient and in-patient services. In Tunbridge Wells there are out-patient clinics where arrangements can be made if required for admission to the Royal London Homoeopathic Hospital.

Homoeopathy within the NHS is also available from some general practitioners. Doctors willing to prescribe this form of medicine can do so on NHS prescription forms where appropriate. But a word of caution here! The standard-sized bottles of homoeopathic medicines that most people use at home are often cheaper than the current NHS prescription charge and many of them can be bought without medical authorization.

There are also many private practitioners offering advice on homoeopathic medicine. For doctors with qualifications registerable for medical practice in the UK additional training in homoeopathic medicine is offered by the Faculty of Homoeopathy. This organization was incorporated by an Act of Parliament in 1950 and is the professional body for homoeopathic doctors. It has its main office in London but operates throughout the UK and organizes homoeopathic courses for doctors in many centres. Postgraduate examinations for doctors are conducted by the Faculty. These are the MFHom and FFHom, the Membership or Fellowship of the Faculty of Homoeopathy.

Many of the doctors who practise homoeopathic medicine work outside the NHS either privately in their own premises or in the increasing number of private or charitable trust clinics operating in various parts of the country. The names and addresses of doctors offering homoeopathic medicines throughout the UK can be obtained from:

The British Homoeopathic Association,
27a Devonshire Street,
London W1N 1RJ.

There are also many non-medically qualified practitioners of homoeopathy in the UK. At the time of writing this, June 1989, there is no single standard of accreditation required for lay homoeopaths practising within the UK.

In addition to this range of sources for advice on homoeopathic prescriptions, there is wide scope for self-help. There are many books available today offering advice on ways of using homoeopathic medicines for self-help for a wide range of medical needs. They can be an important aid to people seeking to find ways of improving their own health.

Having considered diseases for which homoeopathy may be helpful and where it can be obtained we come now to the third question posed: how does it work?

Hahnemann's copious writings frequently refer to his continued probing of this important question. They show how he steadily clarified his ideas of how energies exposed in medicines by dilution and succussion, that is by potentization, interact with subtle energies in the human body contributing to or even causing disease. He naturally applied terms familiar in his day and therefore referred to medicinal energies interacting with the 'vital force', a phrase then widely used to imply unseen energies believed to determine the organic function.

Today we can pursue similar ideas using modern terminology and supported by the ongoing understanding of forces that continually operate within the human body determining its structure and function. It is much easier now than would have been likely in Hahnemann's era to think of energy interactions as the basis of human function. In physics classes many of us have learnt that all matter is composed by energy behaving in a manner that makes it appear solid. This means that our bodies are energy fields with their organic structure and appearance constantly formed by specific energic patterns. We also know from personal experience that there are various qualities of such energy. For instance, we distinguish the processes of thought and various types of feeling or emotion by recognizing their distinct characteristics.

Studies from psychology refer in various ways to the understanding of 'three-part man'. That is, that in any activity we perform there are three basic aspects. These three aspects are thought, feeling and physical application. Or putting it another way, in all physical activity we are able to feel its effects sensitively and assess them in our thoughts rationally. We might refer to this generally today as the psycho-somatic or body–mind interaction. Whatever terms we use, we are describing a continual interfunction of thought, feeling and physical expression.

The effects of a sudden fright illustrate this interaction. The idea of threat, for instance if someone afraid of snakes sees one slither past, is associated with a surge of emotion and a related change in the body chemistry that affects the heart and circulation. Biologists have demonstrated the release of adrenalin in such situations and have termed it the 'fright and flight reaction'. It is a dramatic illustration of an interaction that occurs in all moments, not only those of particular stress.

With this illustration in mind it is easier to begin to understand that thoughts or feeling can change our body chemistry, and going a stage further in our deductions, that psychotherapy, relaxation and related techniques, can help us redirect mental and physical energies in ways that can assist healing.

Hahnemann's deductions on how homoeopathic medicines work correlate closely with such insights. He referred to homoeopathic medicines suitably stimulating the vital force to provoke its opposition to the similarly unseen causes of disease effects. A modern interpretation of his suggestions is that homoeopathic medicines interact with the psychological aspects of the human body and through these help correct the personal chemistry that contributes to physical changes in disease. We might also argue further that Hahnemann's deductions that homoeopathic medicines stimulate opposition from the vital force to assist recovery, correlate with modern theories of immune reactions and their role in restoring health. The response that Hahnemann argued occurred in the vital force in opposing the homoeopathic stimulus can be compared to discoveries of antibodies provoked to counteract an antigen, a disease-causing agent.

Hahnemann's observations about the effects of homoeopathic medicines are today receiving increasing support from various researchers, amongst them physicists, veterinary surgeons and physicians. Some physicists are researching energy patterns conveyed in the high-potency solutions where the dilution and succussion has progressed to a level beyond that where a molecular presence is usually acknowledged. Studies from veterinary practices have given statistics endorsing the benefits of homoeopathic medicines in problems as various as dogs with kennel cough, pigs aborting and cows developing mastitis. And in addition to this, from human medicine there have been studies with disorders as diverse as hay fever and rheumatoid arthritis, showing the benefits of homoeopathic medicines.

All these studies co-operate in probing the effect of homoeopathic medicines. While physicians and veterinary surgeons demonstrate its occurrence, physicists probe its nature and psychologists discuss its dynamics.

It is important work with far-reaching implications, not only for all aspects of medical care but also for the ongoing search for increased self-understanding. Many philosophers and other thinkers, including Hahnemann, have reminded us of the basic need for greater self-understanding. The use of homoeopathic medicines and questioning of their effects can be a continuing aid to this search. First aid can have exciting prospects.

Index